SIT WITH LESS PAIN

SIT WITH LESS PAIN

Gentle Yoga for Meditators
and Everyone Else

Jean Erlbaum

Illustrations by Michelle Antonisse
Foreword by Frank Jude Boccio

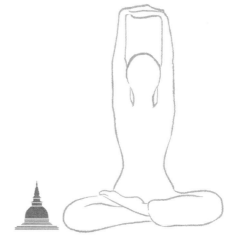

Wisdom Publications • Boston

Wisdom Publications
199 Elm Street
Somerville, MA 02144 USA
www.wisdompubs.org

The practices in this book are not suggested as a substitute for
medical care or advice. As with any new exercise program, it
is best to consult with your doctor if you have any questions or
concerns about doing any of the stretches in this book. Neither
the publisher nor the author shall have responsibility or liability
for any loss or damage caused directly or indirectly from the
information contained in this book.

Library of Congress Cataloging-in-Publication Data
  Erlbaum, Jean, author.
  Sit with less pain : gentle yoga for meditators and everyone
else / Jean Erlbaum ; illustrated by Michelle Antonisse.
      pages cm
  Includes bibliographical references.
  ISBN 0-86171-679-5 (pbk. : alk. paper)
  1. Pain—Alternative treatment. 2. Hatha yoga—Therapeutic
use. 3. Mind and body. I. Antonisse, Michelle, illustrator. II.
Title.
  RB127.E75 2014
  613.7'046—dc23
                                        2013050118

ISBN 9780861716791   Ebook ISBN 9780861716845

18 17 16 15 14   5 4 3 2 1

Cover design by Phil Pascuzzo.
Interior illustrations by Michelle Antonisse.
Interior design by Gopa&Ted2, Inc.. Set in Minion Pro
11.5/16.97.

Wisdom Publications' books are printed on acid-free paper
and meet the guidelines for permanence and durability of the
Production Guidelines for Book Longevity of the Council on
Library Resources.

Printed in the United States of America.

 This book was produced with environmental
mindfulness. We have elected to print this
title on FSC® certified paper. For more information, please
visit www.fscus.org. For more information on our environ-
ment mindfulness program, please visit our website, www.
wisdompubs.org.

To my dear friend, writing mentor, and Dharma sister
Genie Zeiger (1943–2009):
Thank you for your ideas for this book,
which you generously gave to me over your last few months,
and for coming back to sit on my left shoulder
and whispering suggestions in my ear
until it was done.

The mind is like the wind and the body like the sand:
if you want to know how the wind is blowing,
you can look at the sand.

—Bonnie Bainbridge Cohen,
*Sensing, Feeling, and Action: The Experiential
Anatomy of Body-Mind Centering*

Table of Contents

List of Exercises

Foreword

I FIND IT HEARTENING that the postures and movements of hatha yoga are finally being accepted and celebrated by many Buddhist practitioners and teachers. It was not always this way; while today there are Insight Meditation centers—and even Zen centers—offering yoga during their retreats, some younger folk might not be aware that such body-centered practice was often frowned upon or even actively discouraged. In the 1970s, when I began Zen practice, my teacher told me to stop practicing yoga, adding, "Zazen is all you need to practice."

As Jean Erlbaum, who began her practice in 1965, shares, "Yoga was seen as a serious detour from practice." And like her, I found ways to sneak my practice in during retreats: slipping into the woods around the monastery, or doing a couple of standing postures in the bathroom during breaks. Why? Because it works! It helped me then, and it continues to support me now in my sitting practice.

The irony, of course, is that for millennia yoga was simply the practice of yoking body, breath, and mind (the original meaning of the word *yoga*, coming from the Sanskrit root *yuj*, means "to yoke"), which was just what we were attempting while sitting on our zafus. Hardly any of our teachers and fellow practitioners seemed to remember that the buddha *was* a yogi!

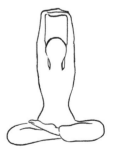

Nowadays, yoga has become mainstreamed and commodified, with an estimated twenty million Americans or more practicing it. The word *yoga* has become synonymous with the postures (*asana*) and movements of hatha yoga, a relatively recent form of yoga, which as contemporarily practiced goes back only to the turn of the nineteenth century, and it has often been divorced from its mental component. Generally, when someone says they practice yoga, what they mean is that they practice postural yoga: the physical forms. But it's helpful to keep in mind that all authentic yoga involves the meditative awareness we cultivate in sitting meditation. When this is understood, the postural practice, as Erlbaum teaches it, "is not separate from meditation practice—it becomes the practice."

I was very happy to see that this is her approach, as it is also mine. In fact, the reason I refer to my practice of hatha yoga as "mindfulness yoga" and not "mindful yoga" is because the emphasis is on the practice of the postures as a vehicle to cultivate greater embodied awareness. The important thing isn't so much that a posture is done mindfully as that mindfulness is cultivated and brought to the practice of the posture. Similarly, Erlbaum writes, "By fully sinking into the specific sensations of each pose, we create the possibility of relinquishing the usual busyness of mind and expanding beyond the usual constrictions of the body, beyond the boundary of 'this self.'"

All this is not to deny or underplay the many well-known physical benefits of hatha yoga for meditation practitioners: from stress reduction and the increasing of the efficiency of the immune system to the relief of muscle and joint pain and increasing circulatory and respiratory health. Who among us practitioners of sitting meditation hasn't experienced sore, stiff, and painful necks, shoulders, or backs? How many of us are free of hip or knee pain or of loss of circulation in our hands or feet? Patanjali, in the *Yoga Sutras*, speaks about preventing the pain that hasn't yet arisen. The practice of hatha yoga can both relieve us from current pain, and with a consistent, well-balanced practice, it can prevent future pain.

In this comprehensive practice manual, Erlbaum offers practical, easily accessible practices, including valuable instruction on proper breathing technique and detailed instruction on a vast variety of stretches and postures that can be practiced on a yoga mat or in a chair. She helpfully presents the exercises grouped for specific areas of the body from the upper body (including exercises for eyes, jaw, neck, shoulders, and upper back) through the middle body, and down to legs, knees, ankles, and feet. I am also happy to see her emphasis on the importance of relaxation as a *practice*. Too many students fail to understand that relaxation indeed requires active cultivation and the time to do so.

In the second half of the book, Erlbaum offers suggested pose sequences of varying lengths—with poses for both mat or chair practice. The sequences are for relaxing or energizing, as well as for targeting specific body "hot spots" of tension, discomfort, and pain. And throughout, she speaks with the compassionate and confident voice of the truly experienced teacher/practitioner who understands the life demands of a contemporary householder. I smiled when she shares having "memories of squeezing yoga sessions into my children's nap times," as I too am finding myself having to continually adapt my practice to my toddler daughter's agenda!

Dogen Zenji refers to zazen as the "Dharma gate of great ease and joy." Too often, for many practitioners, it seems like anything but! This book offers a wonderful resource for yogis who practice sitting meditation and wish to experience greater bodily ease and the joy that arises with it. It is also valuable for yogis with a hatha yoga practice who wish to cultivate sitting meditation; it presents a clear and concise manual on how to create a strong foundation for sitting by using the practices with which they are already familiar. I am appreciative and grateful to Jean Erlbaum for writing this book and to Wisdom Publications for making it available. May it bring great ease and joy to many!

Frank Jude Boccio

Introduction

IN THIS BOOK, I offer not only practical stretches to alleviate tense or achy bodies but also movements that invite the mind to anchor into the body as a form of meditation. Many of the benefits of doing yoga are well known: reducing stress by slowing and deepening the breath; calming the nervous system and relaxing muscles, ligaments, and tendons; increasing the efficiency of all the systems of the body; strengthening the immune system and bringing balance to the whole hormonal system; encouraging the flow of all bodily fluids (blood, lymph, cerebrospinal fluid, etc.). Additionally, deep breathing enhances the work of the digestive, pulmonary, and cardiovascular systems and massages all the internal organs. Many people rely on yoga to prevent or heal back or joint injury, to align and strengthen muscles and bones. Yogis have known for thousands of years that their practices have kept them healthy and strong. As more research is done in the West, the substantiated list of benefits continues to grow.

Yoga has specific benefits for those of us who spend long stretches of time sitting in meditation. There are particular parts of the body that need to be in alignment to stay flexible and strong in order to maintain a comfortable sitting practice. Many folks report achy necks and shoulders, weak middle

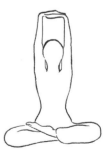

or lower backs, tight hip joints, or excruciating pain in their knees. I have heard some meditators report loss of circulation in their hands and feet, eyestrain, or headache. We each have our weak areas and places we carry stress. The good news is that simple yoga practices can prevent and remedy many of these problems.

One of the most important benefits of yoga is its invitation into the present reality of one's own body: what hurts, what is pleasant, one's particular rhythms of breath and heart beat. In order to be awake, we must not just think about, not just notice, but fully enter into the sensations of knees throbbing and breath moving. Instead of avoiding the complaints of our body, we can honor each sensation as an aspect of our current reality. This allows us to see more clearly the places we hold tight and therefore gives us a greater possibility of wholly accepting and then releasing those places. The path of liberation leads us to know intimately the layer cake of related attachments of body, mind, emotions, habits, and patterns. The stretching and deep breathing of yoga give us an opportunity to recognize and either dissolve those attachments or find skillful means to meet them.

Yoga can bring us into the authentic embodiment of each moment. When we pay full attention during a forward bend, we can drop all memories of how our back has been, judgment of how it should be, worries about how it may get worse, or fantasies of how to make it better. All there is in that moment is the stretch, the breath, and any physical changes or insights as they occur. Yoga used this way is not separate from meditation practice—it becomes the practice. By fully sinking into the specific sensations of each pose, we create the possibility of relinquishing the usual busyness of mind and expanding beyond the usual constrictions of the body, beyond the boundary of "this self."

We can create regular yoga sessions for ourselves and take the visceral awareness this practice promotes into both our formal meditations and into our everyday lives. We can cultivate a larger yoga: an ability to align with our body while sitting, walking, washing the dishes, or climbing into bed at night. We can cultivate mindfulness of what changes with each movement and of the stillness that remains even as we move through our days.

I have been teaching yoga at meditation retreats for over thirty years. The feedback I hear most often is that a body free from tension and pain allows for easier sitting and a quieter mind. Yoga can help us go beyond watching the movements of body and mind; it allows us to become "bodymind," to embody this one thing we always are. My hope is that these stretches help you as much as they have helped me, so that we all can sit deeply and live with grace and flexibility in all circumstances.

Basic Instructions

As you perform the exercises in this book, listen well to your body and honor its limitations. For example, if you have untreated high blood pressure or glaucoma, you may want to skip or modify poses that ask you to drop your head forward; if you have recently had hip, knee, or shoulder surgery, you want to avoid poses that could stress the affected joints; if you are pregnant, there are some poses that are particularly helpful and others you may want to avoid. The model for some of the poses in this book, for instance, is a gorgeous woman named Sojee who modeled some poses in her fourth month of pregnancy and others in her eighth month. She modified the poses as appropriate and used propping as she needed. After the first trimester, depending on the placement of the fetus, many women feel it is best to skip poses that require lying flat on their back for more than a few minutes. Especially after the first trimester, extreme backward or forward bends or spinal twists are not recommended in order to protect the abdominal muscles.

If you have any questions about the wisdom of doing any of the stretches, please contact your healthcare provider or a certified yoga instructor. On some days you may be able to stretch more easily than other days. Please feel free to modify

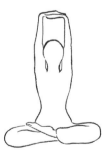

or skip stretches that don't feel right. Experiment with the ways of moving that serve your body. Instead of putting yoga on a list of have-to's and trying to fit in a set amount of poses, allow yourself to thoroughly enjoy each stretch that suits you in each session.

 ## PROPS

Each of us has a unique anatomy, and so it's important to honor our special needs as we engage in sitting or stretching. We may at times have to deal with various physical and emotional discomforts, but there is no reason to endure avoidable pain. For this reason, I make suggestions throughout the book of possible modifications and propping that can support you in a stretch; we can enhance our sitting practice by using props to help us sit comfortably erect. Many yoga poses are possible to do either on a mat or in a chair. If you prefer the chair versions of the poses, please make sure you have a comfortable, sturdy chair. For some poses, a chair with arms works best; in other poses, an armless chair will work better. A wheelchair that is secured and balanced is a wonderful place to practice stretches, using leg and foot rests as needed for poses.

You may want to have the following props handy in case you need them: a yoga belt (or any long strap you have at home), a yoga block, a yoga bolster, a *zafu* (meditation cushion) or folded bed pillow, a small towel, and a flat blanket. During relaxation, you may like using an eye pillow, which is just the right size to cover the eyes and block light. These pillows are usually made from silk, often filled with flax seeds, and sometimes scented with lavender, which is known to calm the ner-

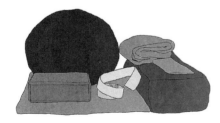

vous system. Feel free to experiment. I have heard reports of great gratitude toward everyday items (e.g., furniture pieces, countertops, couch cushions) as wonderful aids in stretching. Please make sure that the props you use add to your stability and do not detract from it.

 ## CHAIR OR CUSHION: HOW TO SIT

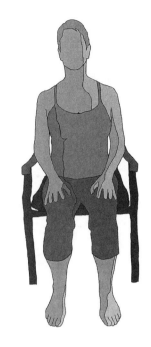

Whether you choose to sit on a chair or a cushion, sit with an erect spine that maintains its natural curves. Your hips should be directly under your shoulders, which should be directly under your ears. Take time to lengthen the back of your neck and drop your shoulders away from your ears. This opens your chest and invites ease of breathing. This kind of alignment provides for a bodymind conducive to sitting. For the purposes of this book, sitting erect in a chair is called Seated Mountain Pose.

If you are sitting on a chair or on the floor, it is helpful to have a cushion under your buttocks in order to tilt your pelvis slightly forward. You may want to use a traditional meditation cushion if you are sitting on the floor and a thinner cushion or wedge if you are on a chair. You can also use a traditional *seiza* bench, which is usually a simple wooden bench, specifically designed for meditation, with this same helpful tilt for the pelvis.

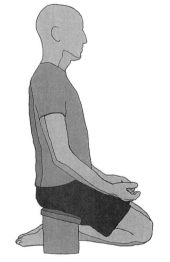

We get no extra meditation points for some kind of "advanced" method of sitting. Experiment and see what allows you to maintain the natural curve of your lower back and to elongate your spine. When sitting

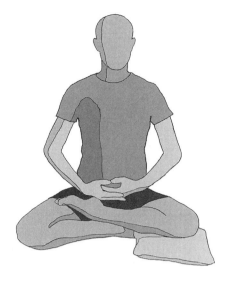

in any traditional pose, try out different props or combination of props to aid affected body parts. For example, in half lotus, placing a small cushion under the knee that is higher will help ground it and prevent strain to the corresponding hip. It is a good idea, if possible, to alternate the leg that rests on top.

If you are in a seiza position (knees bent with legs folded under the buttocks, with or without a bench), raising the height of the bench or cushion you are using can bring relief to lower back, hips, knees, and feet. Feel free to use a pad or folded towel under your feet and knees as needed.

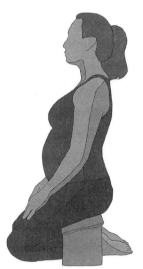
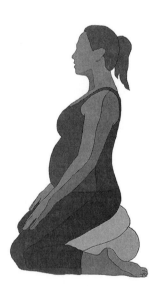

Try massaging ankles, knees, and hip joints at the beginning of a sitting. Try rocking from side to side once you are seated. Being kind to your body on the way into a seated position may make it easier to sit comfortably for a longer stretch of time.

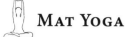 Mat Yoga

Pick a quiet spot with room to move and adequate padding (a firm folded blanket, a yoga mat, or both). Please make sure that the surface on which you are stretching is level. Some of the poses in this book are done lying on a mat and some are done standing. Many are done in a seated position and are possible to do right on your meditation cushion.

Chair Yoga

For those of us with injuries or weaknesses in our backs or knees, it is especially appropriate to sit in a chair when meditating or stretching. Many of us are Westerners unused to floor sitting and may feel more comfortable in a chair.

Many of the poses that are traditionally done on the floor can easily be done in a chair. When there are modifications or instructions for transforming a pose into a chair version, I give special directions for that; otherwise, please assume you can use the instructions on a mat or in a chair. Some of the floor poses do not translate well to chair yoga; for those poses I offer alternative stretches that will give similar benefits. For stability in stretching, you may want to have your chair on a yoga mat or placed next to a wall. For some poses, a chair with arms can give extra support; with some poses, a chair with no arms leaves more space for stretching. Please choose the chair that works best for you in each pose.

If you sit in a chair, make sure your feet and seat bones feel rooted and stable. If you feel a temptation to slump back in your chair, please remember that this disturbs the natural alignment

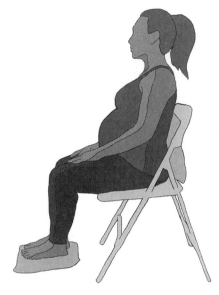

of the spine and, if done as a regular practice, will weaken your back muscles. Please use a chair that is stable, firm, and comfortable. A straight-back kitchen or desk chair will work better than an upholstered chair in helping you keep an erect spine. If you feel your back rounding or weakening, try placing a cushion or a rolled towel between the small of your back and the chair. If your feet don't reach the floor, please place a cushion under them for support.

RECORDING

If you find that you have to interrupt the flow of poses in order to keep referring to the book, you may want to record yourself reading the instructions for a series of poses. This may help the yoga become more of a meditation (instead of a how-to exercise). It may be particularly useful to listen to a recording of the Body Scan and Savasana series while relaxing into the depth of those practices. For information on *Sit with Less Pain* companion CDs for mat and chair yoga, please see the resources section at the back of this book.

STRETCHING

The exercises in this book are designed to release the joints that sometimes make seated meditation difficult and the muscles that tend to get tight in long-term sitting. The poses can be of benefit to overall health, stamina, and clarity. The poses in this book are quite gentle and should be fine for most people, but please keep in mind your own safety and pleasure as you stretch.

Stretching is usually more comfortable when done at least two to three hours after a big meal. An expensive yoga outfit is not essential for your yoga practice, but loose-fitting, comfortable clothes really do make a difference—for example, sweat pants or loose-fitting shorts are great, but tight belts or restrictive jewelry are not so great. For standing poses, bare feet work best as socks or tights can be slippery.

Toward the end of the book, I give instructions for two relaxation practices: one to come before and one to come after your stretching. Please make sure to include these periods of relaxation in your routine; doing so can dramatically deepen the effects of the yoga.

Many people feel that bouncing while stretching will somehow let them get deeper into a stretch. Actually bouncing shortens the muscles and is counterproductive. Once you have found your way into a pose, my suggestion is that you actively rest in it. By "actively" I mean maintaining the edge of your stretch—as far as you can go, which may change as you remain in that stretch—and maintaining your awareness of the moment-to-moment spontaneous shifts of bodymind as you stay in that stretch. By "resting" I mean sinking into the fullness of the stretch without forcing or bouncing. Focusing on the natural flow of the breath and the subtle sensations throughout the body help enhance this active resting.

In most cases, I give directions for just one side of the body and suggest you repeat the pose on the other side. My hope is that the anatomic detail of my words will help massage your body into your best stretch and alignment. Even though I put the poses into separate sections according to body parts, most poses will benefit several parts of the body at the same time. (After all, "the hip bone's connected to the thigh bone…") In fact, when any part of the body is released, the whole body gives a sigh of relief.

Many forms of yoga emphasize a particular alignment for each pose. This is helpful to keep the poses safe, to maximize the stretch, and to build strength. For this book I give only minimal instruction in alignment, asking the reader to focus on comfort, awareness, and release. While there are obvious benefits to focusing on alignment, trying to remember where to place or lift each part of the body can be counterproductive to inducing the embodied, meditative experience that is the goal of this book.

Please allow these stretches to become an integral part of your practice. At the end of the book, I suggest combining several poses into flowing sequences. You may choose to do these sequences on a daily basis to keep your body supple and to prevent injury. And be sure to make note of the stretches that serve you best; you may choose to focus just on the poses that appeal to you as you prepare for or release from sitting.

Breathing

IN MEDITATION, we may count the breath or just watch it move in and out. Often the instruction for meditation is to make no effort to change the breath, just to witness the natural flow of inhalation and exhalation. When we move into yoga, we have a different relationship to the breath because we are using it intentionally in our effort to position the body and then in our exploration of that posture. Usually on an inhalation, the body naturally will expand, lift, and extend. On an exhalation, we can more easily twist, release, and rest.

Breath is said to be the bridge between the mind and the body. It can serve us to slow and deepen the breath and imagine that we are breathing into particular parts of the body as we stretch. Even though we cannot literally breathe into each part of the body, imagining doing so can immerse us more fully in the execution and specific effects of a pose. It can help us to become aware of all the sensations we may find, whether they are pleasant, unpleasant, or neutral. In this way we use the breath and awareness of sensation to enhance the stretching, to keep it safe, and to settle even more deeply into the body.

When we breathe into a stretch, we can visualize fresh blood, oxygen, and energy coming into the part of the body we are stretching. When we exhale, we can imagine that we sweep

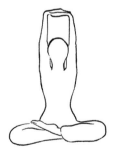

clear that part of the body, releasing whatever we no longer need on the out breath. It is my belief that this visualization of breath moving into and out of the body has very real physical, emotional, and energetic effects; that there is an alchemy created by our physical efforts and our focused concentration. The magic that happens when body, breath, and mind become just-this-one-thing has been known by centuries of yogis and decades of Western medical researchers. We see more and more evidence that full, deep, conscious breathing can maintain elasticity and increased capacity of the lungs, efficiency of the cardiovascular system, and provide a great massage for the other organs as the lungs expand and contract. For meditators, the breath can be used in conjunction with stretching or as preparation for practice right on the cushion. It can become an integral part of one's practice.

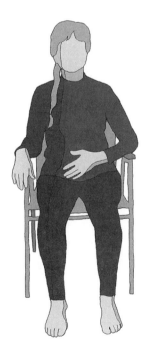

: **Nose Breathing:** Inhaling through the nose (instead of the mouth) can warm and filter the air that comes in, making for easier reception in the lungs. Nose breathing naturally slows the breath and all the systems of the body, including the nervous system. ◾

: **Seated Belly Breathing:** The lower belly, or hara, is considered to be the center of gravity, as well as a locus of power in martial arts. Breathing into the belly at the beginning of a sit can bring focused strength into our practice.

Take time to notice your natural breath. Is it slow, fast, deep, shallow, from the chest or belly, through the nose or mouth? Then, as you feel ready, begin to breathe through the nose, slowing the breath. Placing your hands on your lower belly (as low as you can, just above the pubic bone), watch the belly expand like a balloon on the inhalation and flatten on the exhalation. The instruction "breathe into your belly" is actually an invitation to breathe to the lowest part of your lungs. When we do expand our lower lungs in that way, we press the diaphragm muscle down into the abdominal cavity. This gives the sensation of blowing up a balloon in the belly and creates not only deeper breath, but also a wonderful massage for the digestive organs. Have a few rounds of this belly, or hara, breathing until it feels natural and easy for you.

Many people combine this slow deep belly breath with their meditation practice—whether visualization or koan work or just simply watching the breath move in and out, in and out, belly expanding and contracting, expanding and contracting. This deep belly breath can become a swinging door of inside/outside, self/other, enlightenment/delusion. ■

⁞ LYING DOWN BELLY BREATHING: If it is not easy for you to breathe deeply in a seated position, you may want at first to practice lying down. This can easily be incorporated at the beginning or end of a stretching session or just before going to sleep. Make sure you are comfortable and well supported and on a flat surface. If your lower back is not comfortable lying flat, you can bend your knees, placing your feet six to eight inches apart on the floor or bed.

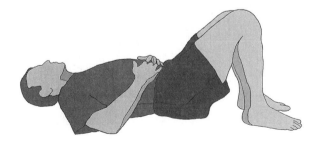

For many people it is more comfortable to place a yoga bolster, zafu, or rolled towel under the knees when lying down. This type of breathing, when done lying on your back, can act as a natural tranquilizer. When this belly breathing is done from a seated position, it can be more energizing, with all the benefits listed above. ■

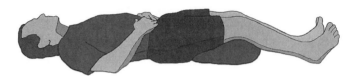

: **THREE-PART DEEP BREATHING:** When you've finished with your belly breathing, you can continue into a full deep breath. Remember to keep your lower back and shoulders relaxed down toward the earth with the back of your neck lengthened, chin to chest. After breathing into the belly as described above, place the hands at the sides of the ribs, fingertips touching, in order to sense the expansion of the middle lungs. Then exhale completely. Please have a few rounds of this two-part breath: belly and ribs (lower and middle lungs), expanding and then contracting.

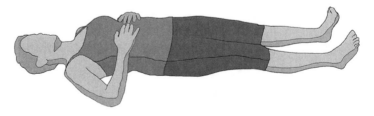

When you are ready for the final step of the Three-Part Deep Breathing, you can place your hands on your chest with your fingers touching your collarbone. In this way you can feel the breath move into the upper lungs, actually raising the collarbone at the top of each inhalation.

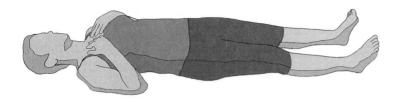

Do several rounds of this Three-Part Deep Breathing: first breathing into the belly, then the ribs, and finally into the chest, holding the breath at the top of the inhalation and exhaling slowly, contracting the chest, the ribs, and finally the belly. Allow the breath to flow in and out this way until it becomes one long, slow, delicious three-dimensional breath. Continue this slow, deep, full breathing as long as you would like.

Practicing this can re-create the habit of breathing fully at all times, which we all did naturally as babies. If done when tired, this Three-Part Deep Breathing can bring us into a deep sleep.

Three-Part Deep Breathing is also possible sitting up. When the body or mind feels unsettled, starting a period of sitting with slow, long, deep breaths can shift us into a calmer state of mind. Using full deep breaths can help move energy from a busy mind into a calmer center in the body.

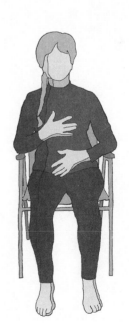

Once these breathing practices become easy while lying down, they can become part of an available repertoire to support our seated meditation. We can use variations of these breathing practices as our needs change. ∎

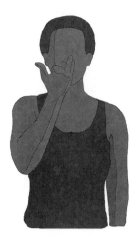

⦂ Alternate Nostril Breathing: If you are feeling particularly agitated, you can do any form of the slow, deep breathing through alternate nostrils. Breathing in this way is said to balance the two sides of the brain and calm the whole nervous system.

The traditional hand position used to facilitate this form of breathing is to bend the index and middle fingers of your dominant hand to the base of the thumb while keeping the thumb, pinky, and ring finger extended. Then use the thumb and last two fingers to alternately close off the nostrils. If you are right handed, you will begin with an inhalation through both nostrils, then close the right nostril with the right thumb and exhale through the left nostril. When you are ready, inhale through the left nostril, close it with the pinky and ring finger of your right hand, lift the right thumb and exhale through the right nostril. When you are ready, inhale through the right nostril, close it off with your right thumb, lift the other two fingers from the left nostril and exhale left. Continue as long as you would like with these slow, deep, alternating breaths, finishing with an exhalation through the left nostril. If you are left handed, please do the same sequence using your left hand and reverse the directions.

If this traditional hand position makes the exercise too complicated for you, please use any hand position that gracefully closes off each nostril in turn. In addition to the physical practice, you may want to add a mental sense of bringing balance and harmony: right and left, in and out, body and mind coming to center. ■

⦂ Rapid Energizing Breathing: If you are feeling unfocused or sleepy, try having several rounds of quick shallow breaths, in and out through the nose with an emphasis on the exhalation. Contracting the abdominal muscles and the diaphragm will help push the breath out and stimulate the hara. Releasing those abdominal muscles will expand the lungs, allowing them to fill naturally and effortlessly with fresh breath and fresh energy.

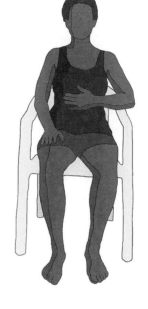

This form of breathing works best in an upright seated position. Rest one hand on your thigh and bring one hand onto your upper abdomen in order to feel the abdominal muscles and diaphragm doing their work. When you feel comfortable with this breath, rest both hands on your thighs to help all parts of the upper body (except the upper abdominal muscles) to remain still. For some of the yoga poses, I suggest using this rapid breathing instead of the usual slow, deep breath. Experiment to see what meets your needs in each moment. Please finish each round of rapid breathing with some slow, deep breathing to bring you back to a calm and hopefully clearer practice. ◼

 ## STRETCHING WITH BREATH

Coordinating each stretch with conscious slow, deep breathing can enhance ease of movement and focus the mind. It is often suggested that we move into each stretch on an inhalation and relax into the pose on an exhalation. I usually recommend then holding each pose for three long slow inhales/exhales. You can certainly take more time in a pose or come out sooner if that's what you need. You can continually rediscover the edge of your stretch using this process of coordinating breath with movement and resting. These practices can keep the mind focused on the subtle mental and physical shifts that each pose creates.

All these methods of breathing can be done on or off the cushion and can enhance the stretching practices offered throughout this book. Once we are comfortable with these breathing practices, the body will naturally use them as needed. We can experience for ourselves how the breath is an integral weave in the fabric of all yoga stretches. We can then let go of any attachment to getting it "right" and move into just stretching, just breathing. It is at this point that the breathing and yoga shift from mechanical, physical activities into a deep meditative practice.

Upper Body

ALL THE POSES in this chapter can be done from a chair, on a yoga mat, or right on your meditation cushion. The illustrations below show some possibilities; please find the form that suits you best.

EYES

Some of us meditate with our eyes closed. Some of us hold a light gaze, eyes partially open. Some of us may sit with concentrated effort; others may have to keep bringing ourselves back from the brink of sleep or mesmerizing fantasies. All these patterns may bring stress to the eyes and to the optic nerve behind the eyes. This can lead to headaches or tired, sore eyes. One simple remedy is a series of eye movements that release the muscles around the eyes.

It is important throughout the following eye movements to make sure that your head stays still so that only your eyes are moving, that your chin stays parallel to the floor, and that you only stretch your eye muscles to their level of comfort. Please remove your glasses (or contact lenses) while doing these eye movements. Before beginning any of these stretches, and between any series of eye stretches, center and then close your

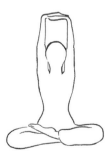

eyes. Take a deep breath and, on the exhalation, imagine any remaining tension leaving your eyes.

: **AWARENESS OF EYES:** Sit in a comfortable, supported position with your spine erect. Close your eyes and take time to notice how they feel. Slowing the breath, bring attention to the area around and behind the eyes, to any differences right to left, and any possible causes of eye strain. ■

: **VERTICAL EYE MOVEMENTS:** Sitting tall, open your eyes to the center of your vision. Slowly stretch them up and down, toward the ceiling and then toward the floor, ten times. When your eyes come back to center, close them and imagine clearing them with a deep breath. ■

: **HORIZONTAL EYE MOVEMENTS:** Open and stretch your eyes horizontally, side to side, ten times. When you are finished, again center and close the eyes, imagining the breath clearing them. ■

: **DIAGONAL EYE MOVEMENTS:** You can also do diagonal eye movements from the upper right-hand corner of your vision to the lower left; then, after resting your eyes, from the upper left to lower right, each ten times. Release your eyes back to center, pause and breathe. ■

: **CIRCULAR EYE MOVEMENTS:** Open your eyes and stretch them up to the ceiling, then continue the motion into a slow, full clockwise roll. As the movements get easier and smoother, you can experiment with allowing the circles to get faster and faster. When you are finished, stop at the twelve o'clock position, close your eyes, take a deep breath, and imagine a feeling of release from your eyes. Repeat the same movement in a counterclockwise direction. ■

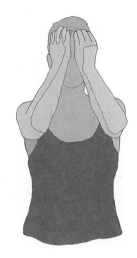

⁞ EYE RELEASE: Rub your palms together to create some warmth and then cup your closed eyes with your fingertips on your hairline, heel of your palms resting on your cheekbones. Again, slow the breath and imagine exhaling out tiredness or tension from the area around your eyes. If you like, finish with some light tapping or massage around your eyes. Allow this to further soothe your eyes and notice any release resulting from the whole series of eye movements. ■

 JAW

When meditating, some of us may follow the traditional instruction to have the tongue lifted to the roof of the mouth and to have lips touching. Even though the instruction is not to hold the jaw tightly, such tension is often the result. Releasing the jaw muscles on a regular basis will help maintain relaxation through the neck, face, and eyes.

⁞ TMJ MOVEMENT AND RELEASE: Massaging the temporo-mandibular joint (TMJ), which is located in front of each ear at the top of the jaw, will often alleviate jaw tension. Sometimes this form of self-massage can also alleviate neck or eye tension or headaches.

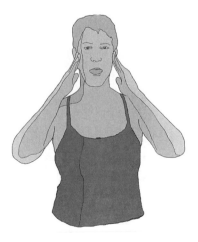

You may want to add movement: open your jaws as wide as you can comfortably and then close them as you continue with strong TMJ massage. Repeat this five to ten times. With your jaws apart, slowly stretch your lower jaw side to side, five to ten times.

Warm compresses can also help if the jaws are particularly tight. ■

Neck

Holding the head erect during sitting can be a challenge, especially if we are tired or have chronically tight neck muscles or any misalignment of the neck or spine. Releasing the neck muscles as part of a yoga practice or on an as-needed basis may be essential. Along with the physical relief, there can be an easier flow of energy between the brain and the body. This often results in a slowing of thoughts, a deepening of breath, and a dropping into awareness of physical sensation.

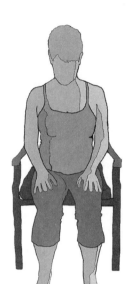

: Neck Stretches, Forward and Back: Sitting tall, lift your shoulders up to your ears, slowly press them back to the wall behind you, and then drop them toward your waist. Maintaining the length of your spine and the width of your chest, drop your chin to your chest, lengthening the back of your neck.

Hold this stretch and breathe along the muscles at the back of the neck. Imagine puffing up the spaces between the cervical vertebrae with each in breath. Let your head drop forward just a bit more on each out breath.

On an inhalation, lift your chin to the ceiling, stretching the front of your neck.

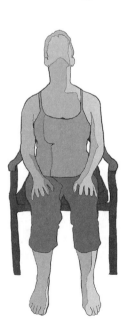

Continue for four rounds with the exhalations dropping your chin forward and the inhalations lifting it up.

Pause at a neutral head position with a long spine and an open chest. Breathe into the length of your neck, front and back. ■

: Neck Stretches, Side to Side: Imagine a string that is being pulled taut from the base of your spine, up and out through the top of your head. Imagine someone near the ceiling gently pulling that string up higher. Maintaining the resulting length in your spine, turn your head as far to the right, then as far to the left, as possible, moving easily side to side, keeping your chin parallel to the floor. ■

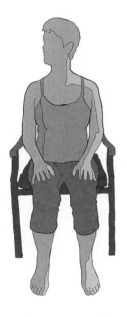 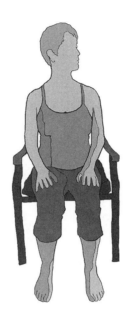

: Neck Stretches, Ear to Shoulder: Beginning with your head in a neutral, centered position, lift your shoulders up, press them back, and then drop them down, maintaining a long spine. Drop your right ear to your right shoulder. Make sure to bring your ear to your shoulder, not your shoulder to your ear.

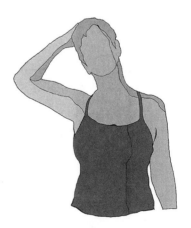

At the same time bring your right hand to the left side of your head, inviting your head further to the right. Bring the fingertips of your left hand to the floor or left side of your chair, next to or just behind your left hip. Roll your left shoulder up, back, and down.

Breathe into the resulting length on the left side of your neck. Imagine that the breath can make the left side of your neck longer.

Release your head and neck back to neutral and breathe slowly, sensing any difference right to left.

When you are ready, do the same movement to the other side. When you feel finished, release back to neutral and breathe into the results, through your neck and through your whole body. ■

 ## SHOULDERS AND UPPER BACK

Sitting straight and holding your arms in one position for long periods of time can bring tension into your shoulders, particularly when, as many do, you have chronic tension or misalignments already present in your shoulders. Many of us carry our "shoulds" in our shoulders, so this area can become a receptacle and a gauge of our mental tensions. There are movements that can oil the shoulder joints and release the muscles and the corresponding attachments. I will suggest a few simple stretches that you can do in a series or singly. They can be done sitting in any comfortable position on a mat or on a chair.

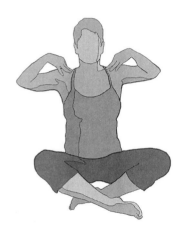

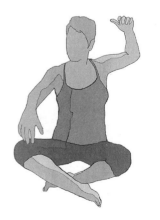

: SHOULDER CIRCLES: Start by sitting tall, putting your hands on your shoulders, and circling both your elbows forward four times. Then circle them backward four times.

In order to make bigger shoulder circles, stretch your arms out in opposite directions, parallel to the floor, with elbows slightly bent. Alternately circle your arms, four times moving them forward as though swimming in a crawl and then four times reversing to a back stroke. ■

⦂ ELBOW/SHOULDER MOVEMENTS: Bring the hands back to the shoulders, point the elbows away from each other, parallel to the floor, breathing fully into the middle back and open chest.

Send the elbows up to the ceiling, stretching the inner, upper arms. Then send the elbows to the floor, pulling the shoulders away from the ears.

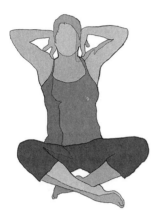
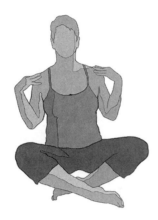
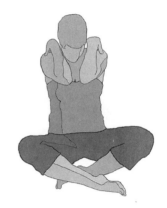

Bring the elbows back to the original position, horizontal to the floor. Bring the elbows forward, toward each other, and lower your chin to your chest, rounding your back. Breathe into the widened back, making more space between the shoulder blades.

To finish the series, roll the elbows back toward the wall behind you, creating a shoulder blade squeeze and an expanded chest. Lift your chin to the ceiling. Expand the lungs even more with slow, deep breathing.

Repeat this whole series as many times as you want and then rest with arms to your sides, relaxing fully through the shoulders. ■

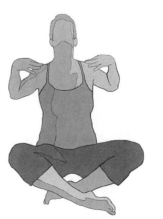

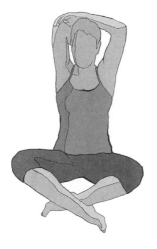

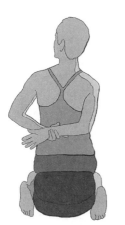

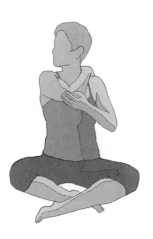

⦂ SHOULDER STRETCHES: From that same tall, seated position, raise your arms overhead. Inhale as you stretch your arms and spine longer, palms facing each other, shoulder joints opening.

Bend the right arm so your right hand falls behind your head and pull the right elbow toward the top center of the head with the left hand. At this point your right upper arm should be next to your right ear. Imagine that each inhalation can make the right shoulder joint more spacious. Exhale out any tension or tightness.

Release your right arm behind your back, elbow bent, forearm parallel to the floor, palm out. Hold the right forearm with the left hand. The right shoulder blade should reach toward the spine. Pull the right arm to the left and look left while dropping the right shoulder down away from the right ear. Breathe into the right side of your neck and down into the right shoulder.

Release the right arm across the chest, bringing the right hand to the left shoulder. With the left hand, press the right elbow toward the left shoulder. Look to the right, squeezing into the right shoulder. If possible, on the exhalation, twist the chin further over the right shoulder.

Rest, breathe into the results, and then repeat the whole series on the other side.

When you are finished, come back to the center with your arms again at your sides. Pause and allow the shoulders to melt down as the spine lifts up. ■

⫶ Shoulder/Chest Series: This series of stretches can further release the shoulders and the upper back. It can also help open the chest, stretch the hands, and strengthen the middle back.

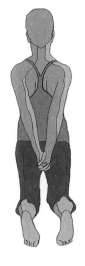

Sit tall in any way that is comfortable for you. Kneeling, with ample padding under your knees, is ideal. If kneeling is not comfortable for you, doing this series from a chair or on a cushion is fine. If you use a chair, please sit toward the front of it.

Begin by rolling your shoulders up and back and then releasing them down. Clasp your hands behind your back, arms straight. Bend your elbows and bring the back of your left hand onto your right hip. Again roll the right shoulder up, back, and down.

Inhaling, expand the chest, and send the right elbow toward the left elbow. Imagine breathing into just the right upper quadrant of your chest as you continue to press your right elbow toward the left, squeezing the middle back, and dropping the right shoulder. After three deep breaths, release your arms to the sides.

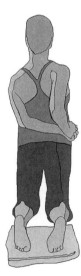

When you are ready, do the same sequence on the other side.

When you are finished, again release your arms to the sides. In order to release more completely, shake your hands, arms, and whole upper body. Coming to rest, breathe again into the shoulders, hands, and front and back of your body, noticing where you have brought some circulation. ■

⋮ LION POSE: This pose is my favorite for releasing shoulder tension and is a great antidote for times when meditation gets too serious.

Squeeze your hands into fists, bring your shoulders to your ears, and make your face as scrunched as possible.

With a loud exhalation, thrust out your fingers and your tongue, lift your eyebrows, and stretch your face. The goal is to look like a scary lion and to roar out whatever needs releasing. Repeat as many times as you want—and enjoy. ■

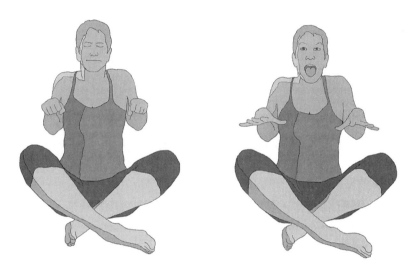

⋮ FINAL NECK/SHOULDER RELEASE: Rub your palms together until there is some warmth between them. Massage your neck and shoulders as strongly as you would like. Finish with light tapping on the top of your head, down the back and sides of your neck, and along the tops of your shoulders.

Please sit with the results of all these stretches and take note of ones you may want to repeat on a regular basis. ■

HANDS

Holding our hands in any set position for an extended period of time can affect circulation to our arms, hands, fingers, and wrists. It can also contribute to tension in the shoulders. In order to avoid these effects and to ameliorate any complicating symptoms of arthritis, we can incorporate simple hand and finger stretches to our daily exercise regime. The following series can be done as needed or regularly each day to maintain flexibility.

⁞ FINGER/HAND/WRIST STRETCHES: Bring your arms out in front of you, parallel to the floor, palms facing down. Alternately, make fists and then stretch the fingers wide for five rounds.

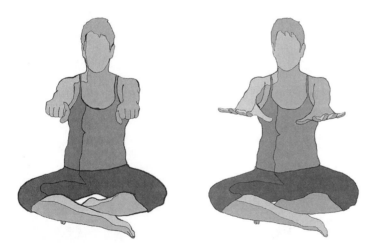

End with your hands in fists and flex the wrists up and down, five times.

Circle the fists five times in each direction.

Stretch your fingers again. Flex the wrists with your fingers up and then down, five times.

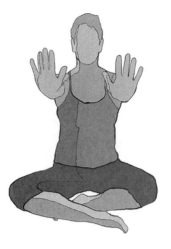 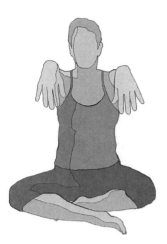

With both arms straight and both wrists flexed, fingers up, dance the hands side to side in an "Al Jolson" movement.

Turn your fingers toward the floor, palms now facing your chest. Dance the hands side to side like windshield wipers.

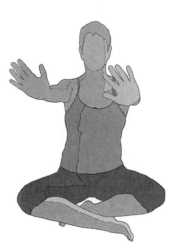 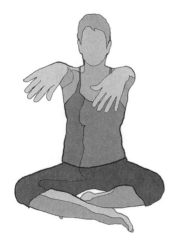

Interlace your fingers and press your palms to the wall in front of you, elbows straight, shoulders dropped away from your ears. Breathe into the arms and wrists and then release.

Interlace your fingers with the other index finger on top and again press your palms to the wall in front of you, elbows straight. Breathe fully into the sensations created and again, release.

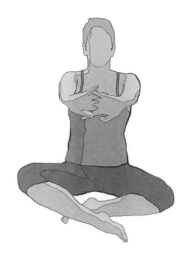

Shake your fingers, hands, arms, shoulders, and head and create further release with a long, loud exhalation. Aaaaah… Rest your arms at your sides and notice the effects on your shoulders, arms, and hands. ■

⦂ ACUPRESSURE ARTHRITIS RELIEF HAND MOVEMENTS: This powerful sequence comes from Lakshmi Voelker's Chair Yoga Series. (See the resources at the end of the book for more information.) It is extraordinary in bringing circulation to the hands and alleviating symptoms of arthritis. Do the following movements thirty-six times, each as strongly as you can.

Start by extending your arms in front with your elbows bent and hands in fists, and tap the thumb side of your fists together.

Then rotate your fists up and tap the pinky side of your fists together.

Now rotate your fists so that they face each other and tap the insides of your wrists together.

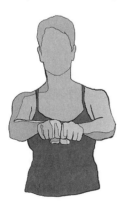
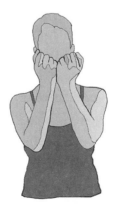
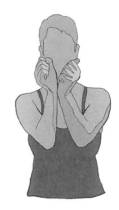

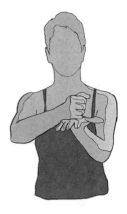

Stretch one hand open and rotate it so that its palm is facing the ceiling. Tap the inside of that palm with the pinky side of other fist. Then reverse the hands and tap again.

Stretch both hands open and tap the webbing between the thumb and forefinger of one hand into the other, and then reverse. (If pregnant, please skip this step; Lakshmi reports that stimulating the pressure point at the thumb web can bring on premature contractions.)

Keeping the hands wide open, interlace the fingers and tap the base of the fingers strongly, one hand into the other. Pause, interlace again, this time with the other index finger on top, and tap.

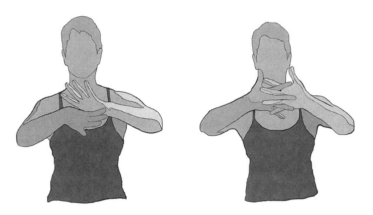

Place your hands, palms up, onto your lap and notice any changes, especially the sense of warmth and circulation in your hands. ■

Mid-Body

O UR SPINE, middle back, lower back, and hips take a big toll in long-term seated meditation. The poses offered below can help release tight muscles and joints and strengthen the structures that help us sit comfortably. Some of the poses in this chapter can be done either on a chair or on a yoga mat just as they are described. The chair poses that need different or extra directions are shown in the following chapter.

 ## Spine

There are many spinal twists offered throughout the different sections of this book. Each spinal twist can offer wonderful benefits: releasing tight back muscles, massaging the internal organs and the spinal nerves, bringing fresh blood flow to the spinal discs, releasing neck and shoulders. Here I would like to offer a simple twist that can be done just before or after meditation. Also offered is a variation that adds an additional release for the neck and eyes.

If you know that you have any problems with your spinal discs, you may want to check with your healthcare provider before doing twists. Doing the poses in a chair, as shown in the following chapter, may allow you to create your own twist modification.

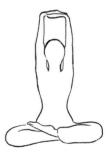

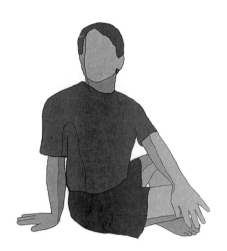

⁝ Simple Spinal Twist on a Mat: Sit firmly on a flat surface in any way that feels comfortable and allows you to feel rooted and balanced through your seat bones. You may want to sit cross-legged, in a seiza position, or have your legs stretched out in front of you.

Inhale, lengthen your spine, and bring your left hand to your right knee and your right hand behind your back to the floor. Turn your right fingers to face the wall behind you and roll your right shoulder up, press it back, and melt it down.

On the next exhalation, start twisting your hips to the right, and then continue turning your chest, right shoulder, chin, and eyes to the right. When you have gone as far as possible, take three deep breaths, lengthening on each inhalation and twisting further to the right on each exhalation. When you feel finished, unwind back to center.

Take time to breathe along your spine and take note of any effects through your body, especially any difference in sensation, right to left.

When you are ready, repeat this on the other side.

When you feel finished, unwind back to center. Again take time to breathe along your spine, neck, and shoulders, and take note of any ripple effects through your body. ◼

⁝ Spinal Twist with Neck and Eye Stretch on a Mat: This is a more complicated but very effective twist that offers an additional release for the neck and eyes.

Remove your glasses, if you wear them, and sit firmly on a flat surface in any way that feels comfortable and allows you to feel rooted and balanced through your seat bones. Inhale, lengthen your spine, bring your left hand to your right knee, and place your right hand behind your back. Turn your right fingers to face the wall behind you and roll your right shoulder up, press it back, and melt it down.

On the next exhale, start twisting your hips to the right, and then continue turning your chest, right shoulder, chin, and eyes to the right. On each inhalation, extend your spine. On each exhalation, twist a bit further to the right.

When you have gone as far as possible, keep the torso in this twist and begin to move the head from side to side, keeping the chin parallel to the floor, looking to the right and then to the left.

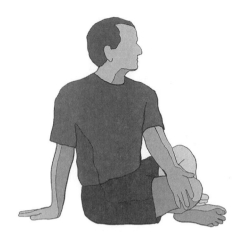

While continuing to turn the head in this way, begin to send your eyes in the opposite direction of your chin. When your chin moves to the right, your eyes move to the left; when your chin moves to the left, your eyes move to the right.

After several rounds of these eye/neck stretches, turn your head to the right and allow your eyes to follow to the right.

See if you can twist even further to the right through every part of your body, again inhaling while lengthening the spine and exhaling into the twist.

After at least three deep breaths, come back to center and breathe up and down your spine and along your neck and shoulders and around your eyes. Please take note of any effects, especially any difference in sensation, right to left.

When you are ready, please repeat this twist to the other side.

When you feel finished, come back to center and again breathe up and down your spine, along your neck and shoulders and around your eyes. You may want to cup your eyes and then massage your neck and shoulders, absorbing the effects of this series. ■

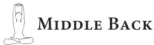 ## MIDDLE BACK

Weak back muscles make it difficult to maintain an erect seated position. Many of us spend hours sitting at a desk or computer and tend to slump when we get tired. The space between the shoulder blades can get tight or achy and can even weaken further as we slump more and more.

We often manifest feelings of sadness or disappointment with a rounded back and a caved-in chest. Some of us chronically protect our heart in this way.

Sometimes the very act of opening the chest and filling our lungs with fresh oxygen can lighten our mood. Most of us need a conscious daily practice of noticing posture, thoughts, and their relationship in order to change chronic patterns. There are several antidotes we can apply as part of a regular stretching practice or at times when we need immediate relief.

: **ROUNDING AND ARCHING ON A MAT:** On an exhalation, hug yourself and bring your chin to your chest. Rounding your back, pull your shoulder blades forward and apart.

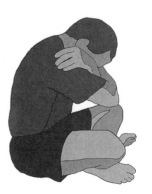 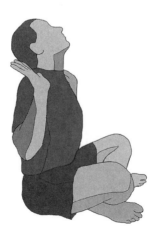

On an inhalation, reverse the position by sending your elbows back behind you, squeezing your shoulder blades together, opening your chest, and lifting your chin up. Continue forward and back, rounding forward on the exhalation, opening your chest on the inhalation.

If you would like to take this further (and if it does not make you feel lightheaded), try rounding forward to hug your knees or even touch the floor.

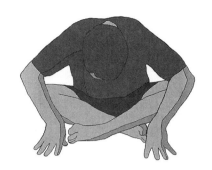

In order to arch further back, bring your hands to the floor behind your back, fingers reaching for the wall behind you, lifting your chest and chin toward the sky.

In whatever version of this series you prefer, enjoy ten series of rounding and arching, bringing fluidity to the spine. ■

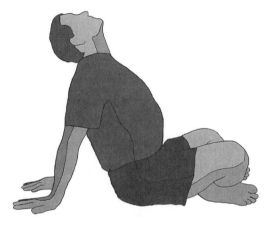

: MIDDLE BACK SQUEEZE ON A MAT: After the last inhalation of Rounding and Arching on a Mat, keep your elbows bent and facing the floor, with your fingers facing the ceiling and palms facing forward. (Your arms in this formation will make the shape of a *W*.) Press your elbows toward each other behind your back ten times, so your shoulder blades squeeze toward each other and your chest opens.

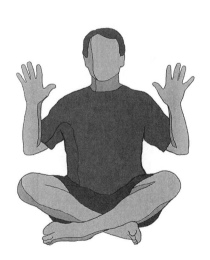

Release your hands to your lap; roll your shoulders up, back, and down.

This Middle Back Squeeze can align and strengthen the spine. It's great for those of us who tend to slump and is very beneficial to do throughout the day, especially when we're doing a lot of sitting, either at a desk or in meditation. ■

HEART / MIDDLE BACK BREATH ON A MAT: After this rounding and arching, you may want to experiment with breathing in from the space between your shoulder blades and out through your heart center. Then reverse the breathing to move in through your heart center and out through your back. Try sounding out loud on the exhalation, imagining as you breathe out that you can release whatever physical or emotional baggage that had been stored there. ∎

COBRA POSE ON A MAT: For those of us comfortable lying on the floor, classic Cobra Pose is a wonderful way to release the upper and middle back, shoulders, and chest. It also provides an internal massage for the lungs, the heart, and the digestive system.

On a well-padded surface, lie down on your belly, with your legs together, toes pointed to the wall behind you, arms to your side, and with your face turned and resting on one cheek.

Anchor yourself to the floor through your pubic bone, thighs, and the tops of your feet. Lengthen your lower back by stretching your tailbone toward the wall behind you.

Bring your palms to the floor under or just forward of your shoulders. Touch your elbows to your sides and rest your forehead on the floor.

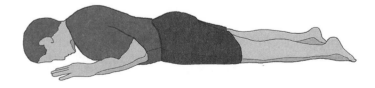

On an inhalation, slowly lift your forehead, nose, chin, and chest as high as you can with comfort, keeping your head in line with your spine. Most people need to keep their elbows bent to make sure the work is being done by the back muscles and not the arms. This pose should open your chest and allow for a gentle backward bend of the upper spine.

Roll your shoulders back to the wall behind you and down away from your ears. Creating a bit of a shoulder blade squeeze and lifting through the breastbone can invite fuller and deeper breath. Keeping the elbows in toward the ribs and the ribs soft will help ensure there is no compression in the lower back.

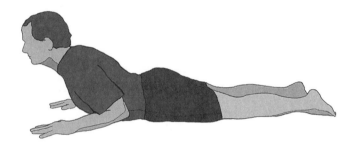

If this creates any stress to your hands or wrists, please keep your forearms on the floor while maintaining the lift through your breastbone. Modify the pose so that it works for your body, and hold it as long as it is serving you. ■

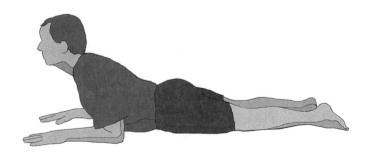

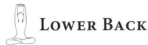 ## LOWER BACK

Sitting for long periods can put quite a bit of strain on the lower back, especially if there is weakness in either the muscles there or in the abdomen. Offered below are poses that are helpful in strengthening the lower back and abs and several stretches to release lower back achiness.

: **CHILD POSE ON A MAT:** The goal of this pose is to create a stretch through the lower back, which was working so hard in Cobra. The name of the pose comes from the position in which many children sleep. Allow your body to be that relaxed in the pose.

As you come out of Cobra Pose, please keep your hands under your shoulders and press your hips to your heels, bending your knees to move into Child Pose.

You can keep your legs and feet parallel, about hip width apart, or if you prefer, bring your knees further apart and have your big toes touching so that your lower legs form a *V*.

You can enhance this stretch with light tapping or massage along your lower back and hips.

If your knees find it difficult to bend in this way, please put a cushion between your calves and thighs or rolled socks behind each knee joint. If the tops of your feet feel too much pressure in this pose, you can put a folded towel or blanket under them.

Some folks like resting in the pose with arms stretched behind the body.

You can also rest in this position with your arms stretched out to the wall in front of you.

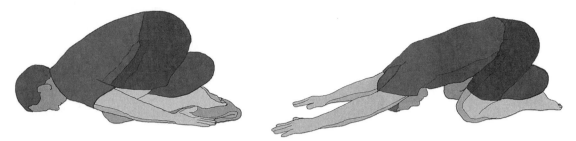

If your forehead does not easily come to the floor, try bending your elbows and bringing one fist on top of the other, creating a pedestal on which to rest your forehead.

Another way to make this truly a resting pose is to place a bolster between your knees and rest your cheek to the side on the bolster. Add more bolsters (or cushions or bed pillows) if you want more height. ■

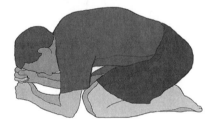
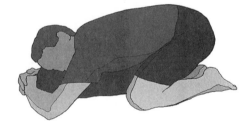

⁝ LEG RAISES ON A MAT: Lie on your back with your knees bent and your feet on the floor. Extend your arms toward your feet, palms on the floor next to your hips. Anchor yourself well through your lower back and shoulders.

Extend your right leg along the floor and point the right toes toward the wall in front of you.

On an exhalation, flatten your abdomen. On the next inhalation, slowly raise your right leg toward the ceiling. Use your abdominal muscles for the lift and keep your toes pointed.

Count slowly as you raise your leg. It should take a count of five to bring your leg from the floor to straight up to the ceiling. Flex the foot and hold this position for a count of five.

On the next exhalation, keeping the foot flexed, lower the leg for a count of five until it is one inch above the floor. Pause for a count of five, point the toes, and repeat the whole process two more times.

When you are done, extend the left leg out to meet the right. Roll both legs side to side on the mat and take some time to rest.

When you are ready, repeat this slow and conscious lifting and lowering with the left leg for three rounds. Please do all the moves with a sense of control through the lower back and abdominal muscles. Roll and rest your legs again when you finish the series.

As these core muscles get stronger, you may be able to lift your straight arms off the floor to more fully engage the abdominal muscles as you lift and lower the legs. You may also be able to increase the number of lifts and possibly even move on to double leg raises. ■

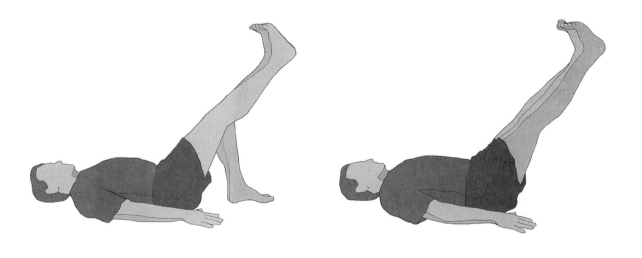

⁞ LOCUST SERIES: This series of backward bending poses, ranging from quite gentle to fairly strenuous, are all helpful in strengthening, stretching, and releasing the lower back. For these poses, you may want to have extra padding under your hipbones.

Begin lying on your belly, arms stretched out to the wall in front of you, toes and tailbone reaching to the wall behind, forehead to the floor. Press the pubic bone down toward the earth in an effort to lengthen and strengthen the lower back.

Reach the right arm and left leg even further and lift them as high as you can. At the same time, if you can, also lift your head and chest, continuing to anchor the pubic bone and reaching with the lifted limbs. Lift your belly button to the ceiling and pull up on the perineum, engaging the core muscles. Hold for at least three deep breaths.

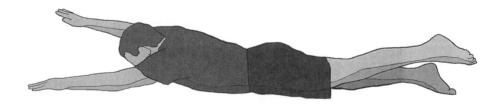

Slowly release down and reverse: lift the left arm, right leg, head and chest, and belly button and perineum. Hold this pose for at least three deep breaths. When you release, rest your head to the side and bring awareness to your breath and heart rate.

If your lower back is strong enough, try a variation of the pose lifting both arms and both legs, as well as the head and chest.

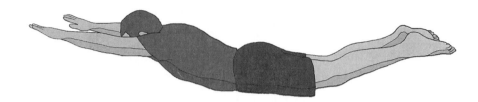

While you lift your limbs, again lift the abdominal muscles and the perineum, establishing core strength for the whole body. When you release, rest this time with your head turned to the other side, again aware of the breath and heart rate slowing down.

For a somewhat more strenuous version of Locust, start again on your belly, this time with arms and legs reaching to the wall behind and your chin to the floor.

Turn the palms of your hands to the floor and lift the right leg, first to the wall behind and then to the ceiling, keeping the knee straight. Hold for three deep breaths.

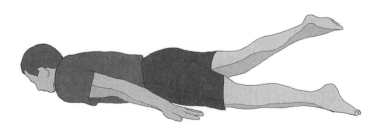

Float the right leg down and lift the left leg, first to the wall behind and then to the ceiling. Hold for three breaths and then rest with the head to the side. When resting after each version of Locust, please alternate the cheek on which you rest.

If you would like, attempt lifting both legs at the same time, keeping the backs of your hands pressed to the floor, your chin to the floor, and your legs reaching first to the wall behind and then to the ceiling, knees straight. Take time to breathe into this pose and then rest, cheek to the other side, shoulders and lower back releasing down.

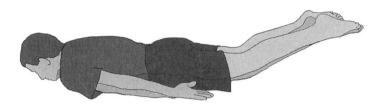

Finally, if you feel you have the lower back strength, repeat the pose lifting both legs and arms to the wall behind, with elbows and knees straight, palms facing the ceiling. You may want to keep your chin on the floor or lift the head and chest. Again lift the abdominal muscles and the perineum. Hold and breathe into the power of the lower back, the lifted limbs, and the core strength sustaining the pose.

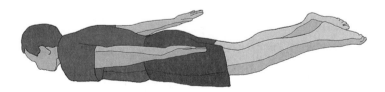

Please take time to rest in Child Pose, releasing the lower back muscles that just worked so hard. Watch the breath and heart rate come back to normal. ▪

: **BRIDGE POSE:** This pose, and the preparatory pelvic lifts that lead up to it, are wonderful for strengthening lower back muscles. Bridge Pose also strengthens the quadriceps, the front thigh muscles, as well as the knees and feet. It offers a backward bend of the spine and an expansion of the chest.

Because the traditional pose is quite strenuous, I will offer several modifications. Please take special care if you have weakness or misalignment through your knees, hips, or lower back. Listen well to your body and go into the version of Bridge Pose that feels best to you.

Begin on your back, hugging your knees to your chest. Keeping your knees bent, place your feet on the floor, parallel, about hip width apart (about four inches for most people). Lengthen your arms toward the wall in front of you, palms down next to your hips.

Start with your hips on the floor. On an exhalation, tilt your pelvis by lifting your tailbone, at first just half an inch off the floor. On each inhalation, lower your tailbone back to the floor. Slowly increase the height of your tailbone on each exhalation.

Continue this sequence until your hips are as high as they want to go. If possible, lift until your thighs are parallel with the floor.

Maintain that lift and walk your feet toward your head until your heels are right under your knees. Press your feet into the earth and lift your chest toward your chin.

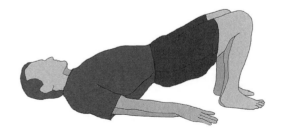

Support the lifting of your hips with one of several hand positions. You may want to have your palms against the floor next to your hips or your hands clasped under your back, reaching toward your heels. If you can, take hold of your ankles, which can help lift your hips and place your weight higher on your shoulders.

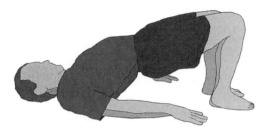 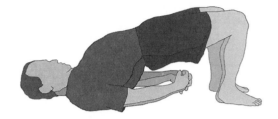

If you feel weakness in your hips or lower back, you may want to use some extra support in the pose. One option is to rest your hips on a yoga block: position the yoga block upright on its smallest end so it stands tall, and prop it under your lower back. You can also support your hips with your arms; press your elbows to the floor and place your hands under your hips, lifting them.

In whatever version of Bridge Pose you have settled, please maintain the lift of your hips and keep the thighs and inner feet parallel, heels as close to under the seat bones as possible. Press your arms and shoulders to the floor and lengthen your neck. At least three times, breathe deeply into the stretch on the front of your thighs and the expansion of your ribs.

When you are ready to release, please lower one vertebra at a time to the floor and then hug your knees to your chest. Rock from side to side or massage your back with Lower Back Circles, as described below. ■

: **LOWER BACK CIRCLES:** This is my personal favorite series for lower back release; it provides a delicious lower back massage. If your lower back is sensitive, you may want extra padding, perhaps an extra yoga mat or blanket.

Lie on your back with knees hugged to your chest. This will begin the process of lengthening your lower back and is a simple way to release discomfort in that area.

When you are ready, allow your knees to separate a bit and support the outsides of your knees with the corresponding hands. Imagine making circles on the ceiling with your knees. Both knees move in the same direction at the same time. Experiment with having your knees closer or further apart as you draw these circles.

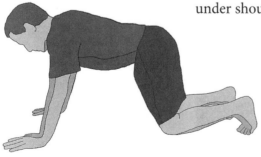

When you are ready, circle in the other direction, receiving a full lower back massage. When you feel finished, again hug your knees to your chest to lengthen the lower back. ∎

: **CAT/COW STRETCHING:** One of the best remedies I know for lower back achiness is a sequence of movements called Cat/Cow Stretching. It is often suggested that these movements be done right after waking and right before sleep to keep the lower back limber.

Start the series on your hands and knees in Table Pose: hands under shoulders, knees under hips with a flat back.

Begin by lifting the head and hips to the ceiling on an inhalation. This is called Cow Pose, because it gives you a sunken spine, like a cow's spine.

On an exhalation, bring the forehead and pubic bone toward each other to create a rounded spine, like that of a scared cat.

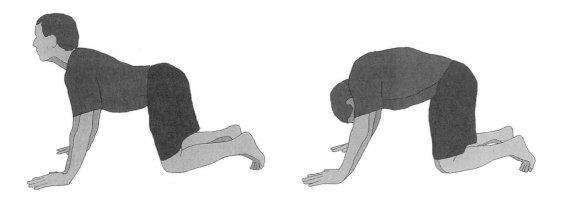

Flow between these two spinal movements, guided by the breath: inhaling up into the Cow Pose and exhaling into the Cat Pose. ■

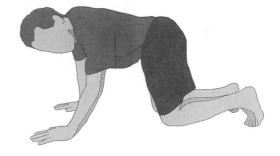

: Wagging Your Tail: Starting from Table Pose, turn your right ear to your right hip and pull your right hip to your right ear; then do the same with your left ear and left hip. Continue to wag your tail, scrunching one side while stretching the other, side to side. ■

: Tailbone Circles: These circular movements are great for releasing the lower back, hip joints, shoulders, neck, and spine.

Starting from Table Pose, bring your knees a few inches further apart. Then imagine you can paint circles on the wall behind you with your tailbone. Start with small circles and let them get bigger and bigger.

As the circles get bigger, place your knees even wider apart and allow your whole body to circle: spine, neck, and head undulating.

After about one minute of big circles, pause and reverse, keeping the circles huge.

After another minute, bring the knees closer and closer, allowing the circles to get smaller and smaller until just the tailbone is circling again.

Coming to stillness, bring the big toes together, keeping the knees apart, and sink the hips toward the heels into any version of Child Pose. Breathe in and out through the lower back, allowing it to release even further. ■

⁚ Knees to Side: This series of flowing movements is recommended for releasing the lower back, hip joints, neck, and shoulders. Do the movements at whatever pace feels good to you. Rest in any aspect of the pose that feels particularly helpful.

Lie on your back and bend your knees toward your chest. Reach your arms out to opposite walls, resting them on the floor parallel to your shoulders, palms facing the ceiling. Allow your knees to flow side to side, going as far to the right and as far to the left as they can.

Allow your head to move opposite your knees in order to create a gentle spinal twist and a stretch for the neck muscles.

Breathe into the massage you are giving to your lower back.

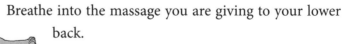

Come back to the default position of knees to chest. Then, keeping your knees bent, bring your feet to the floor, hip width apart (about four inches apart, depending on body proportions).

Again allow your knees to flow side to side, this time with your feet on the floor, moving your knees and head in opposite directions.

As you continue to roll your knees side to side, slowly walk your feet away from each other until they are about 2 to 2.5 feet apart.

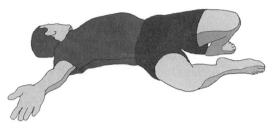

Notice again the massage through your lower back and the additional stretch through your hips.

When your feet are as wide as they will go, allow the knees to come as far to the right as possible. At the same time, turn your head to the left and reach your left arm toward the wall behind you. If your left shoulder complains, you can support it with a small cushion or rolled towel. If you prefer, modify or skip this arm stretch.

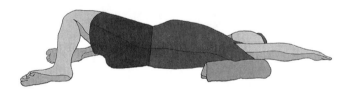

When you find a comfortable position, imagine lengthening your whole left side on the inhalation and melting the left shoulder and hip on the exhalation. Stay in this pose for as long as you like and then do the same stretch on the other side.

When you are finished, have a few Lower Back Circles in each direction and come to rest in any comfortable position, taking time to notice any effects on your neck, lower back, hip, and shoulder joints. ∎

HIPS

One of the biggest complaints I hear from folks who sit for long stretches is about tight and achy hips. For people who sit in any nonsymmetrical pose (e.g., half lotus with the same foot always on the opposite thigh), there is often a chronic imbalance, not only in the hip joint, but a radiation of discomfort through the corresponding gluteal muscles and leg. Any strain in either of the hips can lead to short- or long-term ill effects throughout related parts of the body (lower back to upper back and shoulders, knees to ankles and feet). We can prevent or ameliorate tight hips by paying attention to how we sit (please see the section called "Chair or Cushion: How to Sit" on pages 7–8). It also helps to stretch our hips before and after sitting and in an ongoing yoga practice. There is a series of hip stretches offered below. If you prefer, see the chair versions of these poses in the following chapter.

⋮ LEG OVER, KNEES TO SIDE: The Knees to Side movements (offered above in the section on lower back stretches) can also help release the hip joints. Here is a variation of that series that is especially helpful for hip joints.

Lie on the mat with your feet on the floor, knees bent and close to each other. Bring your arms out to the sides, in line with your shoulders.

Place the right leg over the left, thighs touching.

Slightly shift the hips to the left and then drop the knees to the right.

If you would like, you can add an extra neck and shoulder stretch by turning your head to the left and reaching your left arm to the wall behind you.

As the right leg increasingly weighs the left leg down, bring your breath and attention to the resulting stretch on the outside of your left hip. When you feel finished, hug your knees to your chest, enjoy some Lower Back Circles (page 50), and repeat this stretch on the other side.

After this sequence is finished, repeat the Lower Back Circles in order to release any holding in the hips or low back. Rest in any comfortable position and breathe into the results. ■

: **Goddess Series:** This series offers a stretch and release for hips and knees and a release for the lower back.

Lie on your back, with your knees to your chest. Place the soles of your feet together and allow your knees to drop away from each other.

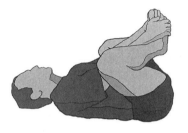

Anchor your head and shoulders toward the floor and invite your feet toward your belly. If you can, wrap your hands around your feet; if your hands don't reach, place a belt around your feet. Please keep your head on the floor. Breathe into your hips, groin, and lower back.

When you are ready, keeping the soles of your feet together, lower your feet to the floor and your knees toward the floor as much as you can comfortably. If this asks too much of your hip joints, try putting cushions under your thighs.

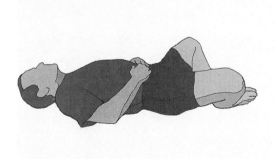

Find a position in which you can rest, perhaps with your hands on your belly to invite deep belly breaths. Stay with the sensations created in each part of your body. ■

: **Hip-Stretching Sequence on a Mat:** As you proceed through this series, one movement should flow into the next for an optimum hip stretch.

If you can comfortably, lie on your back, extending both legs along the floor. Take time to notice any difference from your right hip to the left.

Hug your right knee tightly to your chest and then, using your left hand, bring the right knee diagonally up toward your left shoulder. Bring your right arm to the right and look right. Hold the pose for at least three deep breaths.

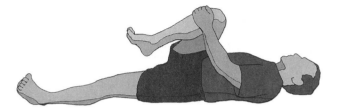

Release the knee horizontally over to the left, toward the floor, and again hold for at least three deep breaths. Please notice how this second movement creates a somewhat different stretch on the outside of the right hip.

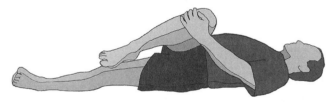

When you are ready, hug the knee again tightly to your chest and then, holding the sides of your knee with each hand, begin circling it with a feeling of oiling the right hip joint as you roll it.

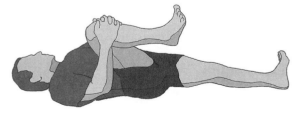

Bring both arms out to the sides and continue circling the right knee, in bigger and bigger circles.

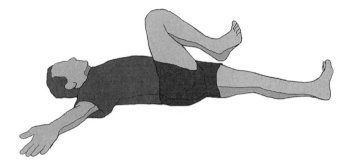

When you're ready, straighten the right leg and continue circling up to the ceiling, all the way to the right, all the way to the floor, and all the way to the left.

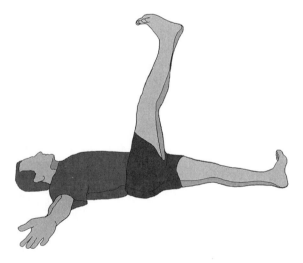

Continue to enlarge the circles and then, keeping them huge, circle in the other direction to the ceiling, to the left, to the floor, and to the right.

Slowly make the circles smaller and smaller. Bend the knee and continue decreasing the size of the circles.

Now move on to the part of the sequence known as the "Knee Down Twist." Hug the right knee to your chest and then place the sole of your right foot directly on top of your left knee.

Inhaling, briefly lift your hips and then roll on to the left side of your left hip, inviting your right knee down to the floor with your left hand. As we have done before, you can add an extra element of stretching by turning your head to the right and stretching your right arm to the wall behind you.

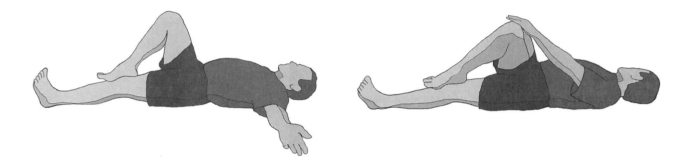

Remember, it is always fine to prop something under your knee or shoulder for extra support, whenever it is needed.

When you are ready to release, move your bent right knee from the left to the right side, with the sole of the right foot along the inner left thigh. You can bring your right foot further down the inner left leg, if that is more comfortable.

Bring your hands to your belly and invite deep belly breathing to melt the hips, groin, and pelvis.

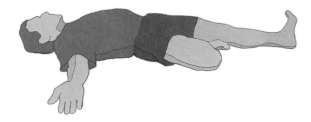

When you're ready, release the right leg straight out to meet the left leg and roll your legs side to side. Notice again any difference right to left and then repeat this whole sequence on the other side.

When you are finished, rest in any comfortable position. If lying flat is not comfortable, try putting a rolled blanket or towel under your knees, to better support the lower back. Please take the time to rest, breathing into your hip joints and lower back and allowing them to melt down toward the earth. ■

: **RECLINING PIGEON POSE:** A somewhat stronger stretch to the hip joints is received in this pose. Please use caution: the more strenuous versions of this pose are not recommended for people who have any injury or misalignment in the lower back or in either hip joint. Also, because one hip is often tighter than the other, it is important to listen well to your body, to do more or less as appropriate each time you enter the pose.

Start on your back, with your knees to your chest. Keeping your knees bent, place your feet on the floor, hip width apart. Please anchor well through your lower back, keeping your head and shoulders on the floor, lengthening through the back of your neck.

Bring your right foot across your left thigh, right anklebone on your thigh about two inches from the left knee.

Press your right knee toward the right.

Reach your right hand into the space you just created between your legs and reach with both hands to hold the back of the left thigh. If you cannot easily reach the back of your thigh with your hands, try using a belt. If you have the flexibility, you can receive more of an opening in the hip joint by holding the front of your left shinbone.

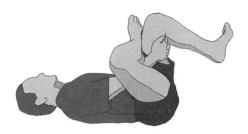

Hug your left knee toward your chest, while continuing to press your right knee to the right. This should create a stretch across the right hip joint.

If you would like more of an opening, press your right elbow into your right inner thigh, flex both feet and shift your body weight slightly to the left.

Breathe into the right hip joint and modify the pose until you find just the right amount of opening.

If you would also like to create a stretch to the outside of the right hip, roll your legs (in exactly the same formation) over to the left, inviting the right knee to the floor with the left hand. You can turn your head to the right and stretch your right arm to the wall behind you for an additional torso, neck, and shoulder stretch.

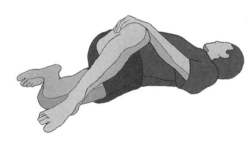

Using your left hand, strongly massage the iliotibial band, which runs along the outside of your thigh, from the hip to the knee. This can help release the attachments in those joints and the tissue between them, all of which can get very tight from long-term sitting. Stay in this position as long as you like and then come back to the knees-to-chest pose with some Lower Back Circles (page 50).

When you are ready, repeat this Reclining Pigeon Pose on the other side. Finish again with some Lower Back Circles. ■

⁞ FETAL POSE: Roll to one side into a Fetal Pose: Resting on your side with your knees bent at ninety degrees with ample support to your head (using your arm or a cushion).

Take time to rest, allowing the whole body to soften, digesting the effects of all the hip stretches. ■

Mid-Body: Variations for Chair

 SPINE

PINAL TWISTS can release tight back muscles, massage the internal organs and the spinal nerves, bring fresh blood flow to the spinal discs, and release neck and shoulders.

Please check with your health care provider if you have any doubts about doing these poses or find discomfort in the poses. If you have a known spinal disc problem, you may want to sit sideways to modify the spinal stretch; if you start the pose in a side-sitting position, you can lessen the amount of twist you take and receive a gentler stretch. When twisting to the right, you can begin the stretch sitting to the right, and when stretching to the left, begin the stretch sitting to the left.

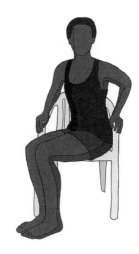

: SIMPLE SPINAL TWIST ON A CHAIR: Start sitting tall with your feet well grounded.

Inhale and lengthen your spine. Exhale and bring your left hand to your right knee or to the right side of your chair beside your right hand. If you can reach easily, bring your right hand to the top of the chair.

Roll your right shoulder up, press it back and melt it down.

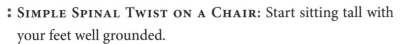

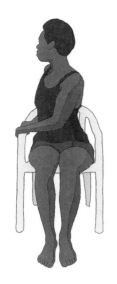

On the next exhale, start twisting your hips to the right, and then continue turning your chest, right shoulder, chin, and eyes to the right.

When you have gone as far as possible, take three deep breaths, lengthening on each inhalation and twisting a bit further to the right on each exhalation.

When you feel finished, unwind back to center. Please take time to breathe along your spine and take note of any effects through your body, especially any difference in sensation, right to left.

When you are ready, repeat this on the other side. When you feel finished, unwind back to center. Again, please take time to breathe along your spine, neck, and shoulders and take note of any other ripple effects through your body. ■

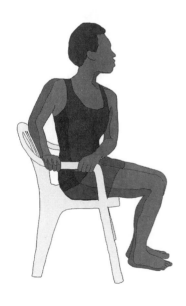

: **SPINAL TWIST WITH NECK AND EYE STRETCH ON A CHAIR:** Start by sitting tall with feet well grounded. Again, if it is more appropriate for you, you may want to sit sideways, facing right on your chair to modify the spinal stretch to the right.

Remove your glasses, if you wear them.

Inhale and lengthen your spine; exhale and bring your left hand to your right knee or to the right side of your chair beside your right hand. If you can reach easily, bring your right hand to the top of the chair.

Roll your right shoulder up, press it back, and melt it down.

On the next exhale, start twisting your hips to the right, and then continue turning your chest, right shoulder, chin, and eyes to the right. On each inhalation, extend your spine. On each exhalation, twist a bit further.

When you have gone as far as possible, keep your torso in this twist and begin to move your head from side to side, keep

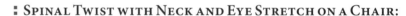

ing the chin parallel with the floor, looking to the right and then to the left.

While continuing to turn the head in this way, begin to send your eyes in the opposite direction of your chin. When your chin moves to the right, your eyes move to the left; when your chin moves to the left, your eyes move to the right.

After several rounds of these eye/neck stretches, turn your head to the right and allow your eyes to follow the chin to the right. See if you can twist even further to the right through every part of your body, again inhaling the spine longer and exhaling into the twist.

After at least three deep breaths, come back to center and breathe up and down your spine, along your neck and shoulders and around your eyes. Please take note of any effects, especially any difference in sensation, right to left.

When you are ready, please repeat the twist to the other side.

When you are finished, come back to center and again breathe up and down your spine, along your neck and shoulders and around your eyes. You may want to cup your eyes and massage your neck and shoulders, absorbing the effects of this series. ■

 ## MIDDLE BACK

Many of us spend many hours sitting in chairs: for meditation, for office or computer work, socializing, eating, watching TV. Some of us spend our days in wheelchairs. And many of us have not figured out a way to do all this sitting without it taking a toll on our body. Unless we have very strong posture or perfectly designed chairs, we tend to feel weak and achy even after a short time of sitting. We develop a habit of slumping, which further exacerbates the problem by weakening the back muscles, contracting the chest, and thereby preventing full, deep breathing. Yoga can help us reverse these long-held negative habits and patterns. In the short term, it can offer relief to our tired muscles.

: **ROUNDING AND ARCHING ON A CHAIR:** On an exhalation, hug yourself and bring your chin to your chest. Rounding your back, pull the top of your shoulders forward and your shoulder blades apart.

On an inhalation, reverse the position by sending your elbows back behind you, squeezing your shoulder blades together, opening your chest, and lifting your chin up.

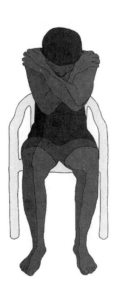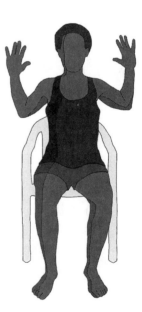

Continue forward and back, rounding forward on the exhalation, opening your chest on the inhalation, for ten rounds.

If you would like to take this further (and if it does not make you feel lightheaded), try rounding forward to hug your knees or even to touch the floor.

In order to arch further back, sit at the front of your chair and reach your hands to the back of the chair. Arch your spine back and open your chest and chin toward the sky.

Repeat the variations you choose for ten rounds each. ■

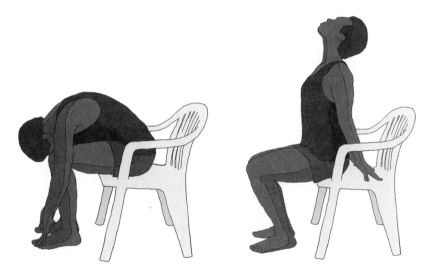

: Middle Back Squeeze on a Chair: After the last inhalation of Rounding and Arching on a Chair, keep your elbows bent and facing the floor, with your fingers facing the ceiling and palms facing forward. (Your arms in this formation will make the shape of a *W*.) Press your elbows toward each other behind your back ten times, again with a shoulder blade squeeze and an open chest.

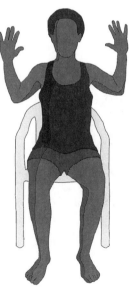

Finish by releasing your hands, palms down on your thighs, and rolling your shoulders up back and down.

This Middle Back Squeeze can align and strengthen the spine. It is great for those of us who tend to slump and is very helpful to do throughout the day, especially when we are doing a lot of sitting. ■

: HEART / MIDDLE BACK BREATH ON A CHAIR: After this rounding and arching, you may want to rest your hands on your thighs and experiment with breathing in from the space between your shoulder blades and out through your heart center. Then reverse the breathing to move in through your heart and out through your back. Try sounding out loud on the exhalation, imagining as you breathe out that you can release whatever physical or emotional baggage that had been stored there. ■

: COBRA/CHILD POSE ON A CHAIR: Please sit in a sturdy chair and place another chair in front of you. The back of this second chair should be about one foot in front of you. You may want to place the second chair against the wall for stability.

Sit tall, hands resting on the top of the chair in front of you. Press your feet down and lift your breastbone up.

Press your hips forward and move into a backward bend of your upper spine, keeping your head in alignment with your spine. Keep your bent elbows close to your ribs, drop your shoulders, and breathe deeply into your chest.

This gentle backward bend of the upper spine is a wonderful way to release back muscles, shoulders, and chest. The expansion it creates through our chest encourages full use of our lung capacity.

When you feel finished, lift to an upright position.

Adjust the front chair so that it is about two feet in front of you. Plant your feet on the floor, fold forward from your hips, and reach your arms to the top, sides, seat, or legs of the chair in front of you. Feel your hands and shoulders stretch to the wall in front of you and your tailbone stretch to the wall behind you.

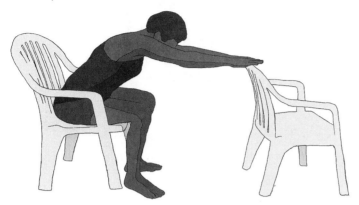

We do this pose to create an opposite stretch from the backward bend of Cobra. We want a good lengthening of all the back muscles, especially stretching the lower back.

Breathe into the lengthening of your whole back and spine. When you are finished, again come to an upright position. ■

 LOWER BACK

⁞ LEG RAISES ON A CHAIR: These lifts are great for strengthening the lower back and abdominal muscles that we use in our effort to sit erect.

Sit in Seated Mountain Pose (see page 7) and hold each side of the chair for balance. (As your core muscles get stronger, you may want to try crossing your arms at your chest instead of holding the sides of the chair.)

On an exhalation pull in your abdominal muscles. On an inhalation, point the toes on your right foot and lift your straightened right leg to a count of five. At the top of the lift, when your leg is parallel to the floor, flex your foot and hold the pose for a count of five.

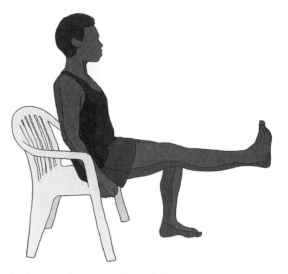

On an exhalation, keeping the abdominal muscles engaged and the foot flexed, lower your leg for another count of five until your foot is about three inches off the floor. Hold this pose for a count of five. On the next inhalation, point the right toes and repeat the whole process two more times.

When you are done, stomp your feet a few times and then take time to rest.

When you are ready, repeat this slow and conscious lifting and lowering on the other side, again for three rounds. Please remember to sit tall and keep your abdominal muscles engaged throughout. As these core muscles get stronger, you may also be able to increase the number of lifts and possibly even move on to double leg raises. Please remember to release and rest your legs when you are finished; sitting tall in Seated Mountain Pose, breathe deeply into your back and belly, feel your core muscles getting stronger and stronger. ■

: **Seated Backward Bend on a Chair:** Start at the front of your chair in Seated Mountain Pose (see page 7). Establish your alignment and take a few deep breaths.

Reach your arms back so your hands can hold the back of your chair seat. If this creates too much of a backward bend, you can either make fists and bring them into the small of your back or rest your hands on your hips.

In whatever position you choose, drop your head back any amount you can comfortably, lifting your chin to the ceiling. Press your elbows toward each other behind your back and take three deep breaths into your expanded chest.

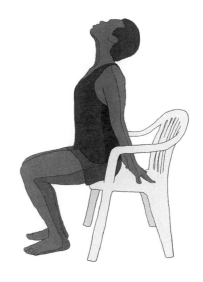

Release back to Seated Mountain Pose when you feel ready. Repeat the Seated Backward Bend one or two more times, holding a bit longer each time, if you can.

When you feel finished, take time to notice the effects through your body and on your breathing. ▪

 Hips

Please begin by sitting tall in one chair and have another chair close by. Use whatever propping you need to feel comfortable. Even before you begin to stretch, take time to notice any difference from your right hip to the left or areas around either hip that may feel tight.

: **Hip-Stretching Sequence on a Chair:** Hug your right knee tightly to your chest and then, using your left hand, bring the knee diagonally up toward your left shoulder. Hold the right side of the chair with your right hand, look right, and breathe deeply into the outer right hip.

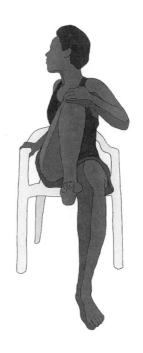

Then release the knee horizontally over to the left, still holding the chair with the right hand and looking right. Please notice how this second movement creates a somewhat different stretch in the outside of the right hip.

When you are ready, you can hug the knee again tightly to your chest with both hands and then begin circling it with a feeling of oiling that right hip joint as you roll it.

Continue circling the right knee in bigger and bigger circles.

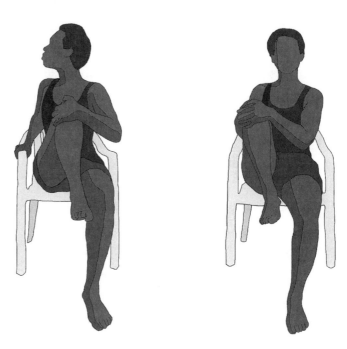

When you are ready, hold the sides of your chair, straighten that right leg and continue circling it up to the ceiling, all the way to the right, to the floor, and all the way to the left.

Continue to enlarge the circles and then, keeping them huge, circle in the other direction, to the ceiling, to the left, to the floor, and to the right.

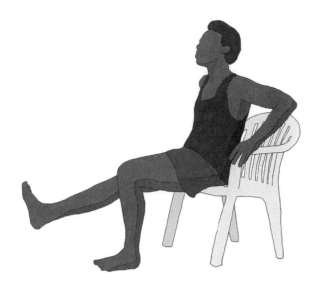

Slowly make the circles smaller and smaller. Bend the knee, hold it with both hands, and continue decreasing the size of the circles. When you are ready to release your leg, come back to center, bring your right foot to the floor and sit tall.

Bring your hands to your belly and invite deep belly breath to melt the hips, groin, and pelvis. Please take time to notice any difference right to left and then repeat this whole sequence on the other side.

When you are finished, allow your whole lower body to sink down toward the earth as you maintain the length of your spine and the expansion of your chest. ■

⦂ **Pigeon Pose on Two Chairs:** A somewhat stronger stretch to the hip joints is received in this seated version of Pigeon Pose. Please note that the more strenuous versions of this pose are not recommended for people who have any injury or misalignment of the lower back or either hip. Also, because one hip is often tighter than the other, it is important to listen well to your body, to do more or less as appropriate each time you enter the pose.

Start by sitting tall on your chair with your legs extended to the seat of another chair facing you. Bring your right foot across your left thigh, so that your right anklebone rests about two inches from the left knee.

While pressing your right knee toward the floor, begin to bend your left knee until you feel a stretch in your right hip joint. You may want to hold the sides of your chair for stability. If you would like more of an opening, press your right elbow into your right inner thigh and flex both feet.

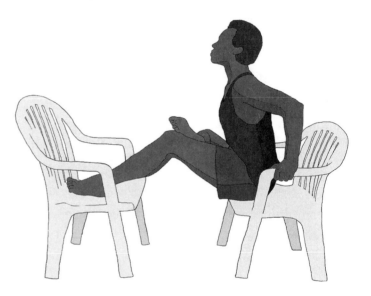

Please breathe into the right hip joint and modify the pose until you find just the right amount of stretch.

Stay in this position as long as you like and then come back to sitting tall with your feet rooted to the floor and your spine long, noticing any difference between the right and left hip joints. Repeat on the other side when you are ready. ■

⁞ BENT KNEE TWIST ON A CHAIR: For a stretch to the outside of the right hip, lift your straight left leg onto a facing chair or keep your left foot on the floor, left knee bent. Place the sole of your right foot onto your left knee and invite your right knee over to the left with the left hand. Hold the right side of your chair with your right hand and turn your upper torso and head to the right.

If you want, use your right hand to strongly massage along the iliotibial band, which runs along the outside of your thigh, from the hip to the knee. This can help release the attachments in those joints and the tissue between them, all of which can get very tight from long-term sitting.

Stay in this position as long as you like and then come back to sitting tall with your feet rooted to the floor and your spine long, noticing any difference between the right and left hip joints. Repeat on the other side when you are ready.

When you're finished, please take time to rest and to notice any further release through your hip joints and through your whole lower body. ■

Legs, Knees, Ankles, and Feet

WHEN WE SIT for long periods, our feet and ankles are asked to remain still, often in somewhat unnatural positions. Many meditators report losing circulation to their feet and legs during sitting. Most traditional meditation positions (except for sitting in a chair) create quite a bit of stress for the knees and their surrounding muscles and ligaments; the knee is the largest and most vulnerable joint in the body because it is both weight bearing and also quite flexible.

Walking between sitting periods is a traditional (and perfect) way to keep our feet and knees released and functioning well. Some of us, especially those of us who sit for days or weeks at a time, need even more attention to our lower body. Yoga can prevent injury by keeping the muscles and joints both strong and flexible.

Please use your own sense of your body to decide which of the following poses are appropriate for you. If you have any known misalignment or chronic pain in your legs, knees, ankles, or feet, please check with your healthcare provider before attempting these stretches. The following series can be done on a mat or on a chair. If you prefer stretching on a chair, have an extra chair near you for some of the poses. The illustrations below show some possibilities; please find the form that suits you best.

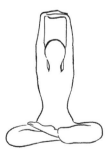

For any of the hip-opening poses, cushions under the thighs may be helpful for people with particularly tight or overly loose hip joints. The model for these poses, Sojee, was pregnant when we photographed her. As you can see, she chose to do several adaptations of the poses. For all of us, pregnant or not, listening well to the body and modifying the poses allow for a happy body and a calm mind.

Lower Body Warm-Up

This series of movements is a wonderful preparation for any sitting position. It works to release feet, ankles, knees, and hip joints. All the poses in this series can be done sitting on a mat or on a chair with another chair facing you.

⁝ **Knee/Hip/Ankle Warm-Up:** Stretch out the left leg to the floor or to a facing chair, keeping the left foot flexed. Bend your right knee and bring the right foot across your left thigh.

Bring your hands behind you (to the floor or to the back of the chair), fingers reaching to the wall behind you. Lean back, creating a slight backward bend of the spine, opening the chest.

Inhale and lengthen your spine; exhale and release your right knee down. Repeat this movement at least two more times. ■

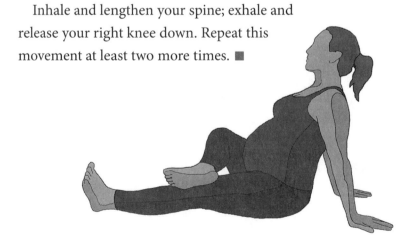

⁚ LEG CRADLING: Lift your bent right leg, bringing the lower leg toward your body. Cradle it by holding the right knee in the crook of your right elbow and cradle the right foot in the crook of the left elbow or in the left hand. Sit tall with your bent leg toward your chest, chest toward bent leg, belly muscles engaged, and spine long. Rock your right leg side to side and then hug it closer to your chest. ■

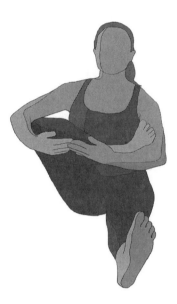

⁚ BENT KNEE CIRCLING: Continuing to sit tall with your right knee bent and your lower right leg horizontal to the floor, cup your right heel with both hands. Begin circling your right knee in one direction and then the other.

Again hug your leg toward your chest while keeping your spine long.

When you feel finished, release the right leg down to meet the left. Roll your legs from side to side. ■

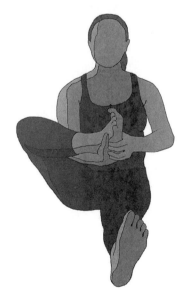

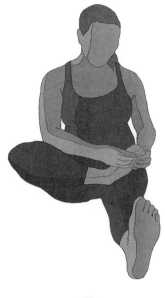

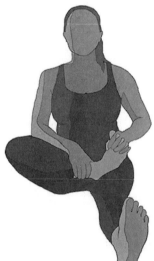

Foot/Leg Massage: Bring your right foot again onto your left thigh. Begin to massage the bottom and then the top of your right foot.

Move on to massage your ankle, heel, and calf muscles. Massage through the lower leg and the front, back, and sides of your knee.

Make a light fist and tap lightly along the outside of your right thigh and around your right hip and gluteal muscles.

With your right foot still on your left thigh, hold your right ankle with your right hand and interlace your left fingers through your right toes and press them forward and back.

Finish by slapping the bottom of your right foot with your left hand.

Allow your right leg to rest in any comfortable position. Please notice any difference right to left and breathe into the results, releasing any tight muscles on the exhalation.

When you are ready, repeat the whole Lower Body Warm-Up on the other side. ■

 ## Knee Stretch and Massage

Because my knees are arthritic, I rarely attend a meditation retreat without making sure I have two ice packs stashed in the freezer. Applying those ice packs to each knee before I go to sleep eases whatever inflammation has occurred and prepares me for the following day's sitting. Some folks prefer heat to bring circulation into their joints. One of the simplest remedies for complaining knees is to massage the front and sides of the joint throughout the day, whenever the knees request some attention.

I would like to offer a variation of a wonderful sequence I learned from Lakshmi Voelker's Chair Yoga Series. (See the resources section at the end of the book for more information on her work.) This sequence can be done sitting on a chair or right on your meditation cushion.

: **ACUPRESSURE KNEE-STRENGTHENING EXERCISE:** Bring both hands behind the right knee, lift the lower right leg and begin to swing it. As you swing, massage strongly on the inside and outside of the knee with your thumbs.

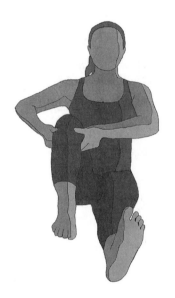 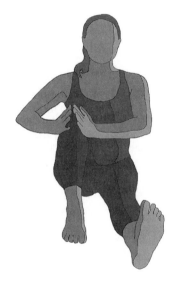 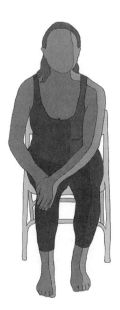

Keeping the knee bent, place your right foot on the floor and massage the inside and outside of the knee with open palms.

Then place both hands, one palm on top of the other, on the kneecap and gently massage in one direction and then the other, in big circles.

Stretch your legs and shake them out. Please take time to notice any difference right to left and then repeat the series on the other side.

When you are finished, stretch and shake your legs again. Pause again to notice the results. Are your knees thanking you? ∎

⁝ STICK POSE: This is the foundation for many seated stretches. This straight-leg position is a wonderful preliminary stretch for the calf muscles and attachments into the knee joint. By tightening the fronts of the thighs and lifting the kneecaps toward the center of the body, we begin to strengthen to the knee. You can repeat this simple movement whenever you like—for example, while standing in line at the grocery store or while waiting for a round of walking meditation to begin. It can bring strength to the legs and alignment through the whole body. Stick Pose also stretches the feet and ankles as well as the hip and thigh muscles we worked on previously.

Sit tall with your legs stretched on the floor or to the seat of a chair placed in front of you.

Flex your feet and lengthen the muscles along the back of your lower legs. Keep your heels pressed toward the wall in front of you, your toes to the ceiling, and the back of your knees melting toward the floor or chair.

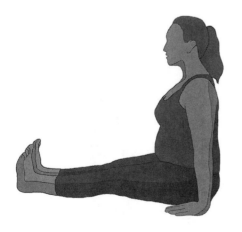

Lift back the flesh of the right buttock with your right hand and then lift the flesh of the left buttock with your left hand. This allows you to sit directly on the sit bones and to lengthen both the hamstring and lower back muscles.

Maintaining an erect posture, engage the core muscles by contracting your belly and perineum.

Place your hands palms down on your thighs, on the floor adjacent to your hips, or hold the sides of your chair.

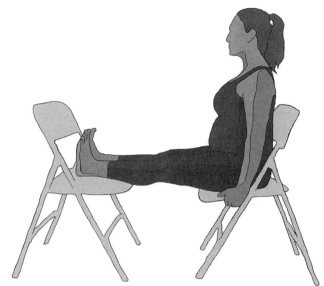

Lengthen in all directions; make as much space as you can between your heels and hips, tailbone and crown of the head. ■

⦂ **FOOT STRETCHES:** Remaining in Stick Pose, rest your hands on the floor or chair next to your hips. If you prefer, bring your hands behind your back, turn your fingers toward the wall behind you, and have a slight backward bend of your upper spine, your chest opening to the ceiling.

From this position, begin to flex and point your feet.

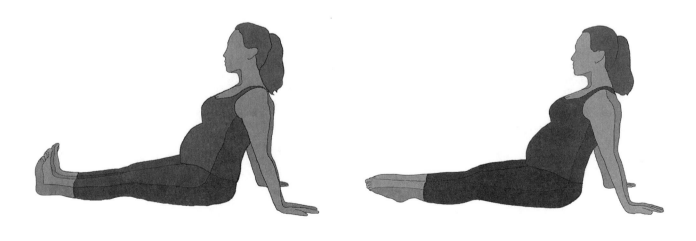

Notice that when you flex, pressing your heels out and toes up, you create a stretch along the back of your legs, from the Achilles tendons to the hamstring muscles along the back of your thighs. When you point your toes, you create a stretch through the front of your legs, from the tops of your feet through the quadriceps muscle on the front of the thigh.

When you feel finished with pointing and flexing, separate your feet a bit and begin to "windshield wiper" your feet from side to side.

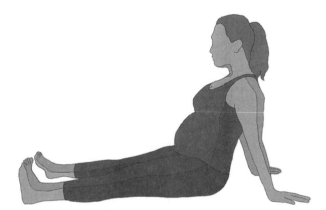 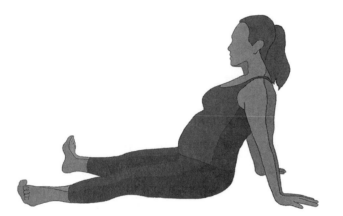

Then separate the feet about a foot and begin to make ankle circles in one direction and then the other. ■

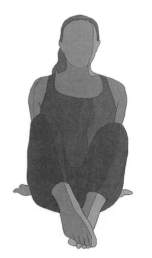

ISOMETRIC FOOT PRESS: If you are sitting on the floor, bend your knees and hug them to your chest, keeping your feet on the floor and your spine erect. If you are in a chair, simply place your feet on the floor close together. Place your hands next to your hips on the floor or hold the sides of the chair.

Bring the sole of your right foot directly on top of the left foot. Press down with the right foot while lifting strongly the toes of the left foot. Create an isometric contraction by equally pressing each foot toward the other.

When you feel finished, release the press, stretch your legs out, shake them, and repeat this movement on the other side. In addition to helping the knees release, these foot and ankle stretches are often a welcome relief after holding one's feet still during meditation. ◼

⫶ Elbow/Knee Press: This series of stretches can be done from a chair or the floor. They can provide strength and also release for the knees, shoulders, and hips.

Sit with the knees bent, feet on the floor, about two feet apart. With your palms together, place your elbows at the inside of each corresponding knee.

Keeping the feet in place, allow the elbows to separate the knees as much as possible, creating a stretch to the inner thigh muscles.

Keeping the feet two feet apart, allow the knees to press the elbows in toward each other, strengthening the inner thighs.

Then create an isometric stretch by equally pressing the knees and elbows, bringing strength to both the legs and arms. ◼

ON A MAT

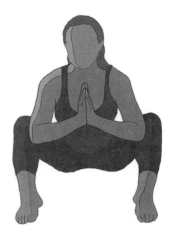

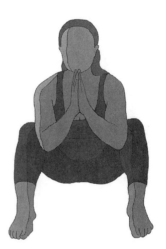

ON A CHAIR

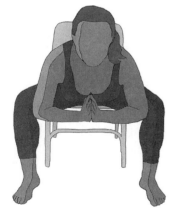

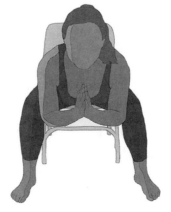

FORWARD BENDS

Variations of forward-bending poses are offered here to give a stretch to all the muscles of the legs. Some variations also stretch the muscles of the back. All variations offer a gentle massage to the internal organs as we fold forward. Modifications of the forward bends can be done from a chair as shown below.

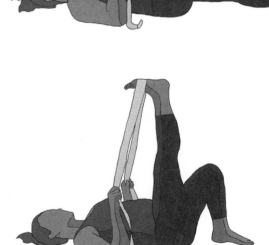

: **LEG LIFTS ON A MAT:** A gentle version of forward bending is achieved with a series of stretches I call Leg Lifts. For these, you'll need an exercise belt. It's important that your belt is long enough to allow you to fully extend your leg while keeping your shoulders on the floor—thereby keeping your chest open and enabling slow, deep breathing.

Lie down on your back on a yoga mat. Your legs may be stretched out to the floor in front of you or you may have your knees bent, feet to the floor. Anchor well through the lower back.

Put a belt around the ball of your right foot and hold the ends of the belt with each hand. Lift the right leg to the ceiling as straight and as high as you can.

Keep your shoulders rolled back away from your ears, down toward the mat. Extend the right leg and flex the foot, heel to the ceiling.

If the left leg is extended on the floor, flex the left foot. If you choose to keep the left knee bent with the left foot on the mat, please keep the left foot, knee, and hip aligned and well anchored.

Position the right leg so that you can keep the right knee straight.

Breathe along the back of the right leg, extending the Achilles tendon, calf, and hamstring muscles. Hold the belt in a way that allows the arms and shoulders to remain relaxed. This keeps the emphasis on stretching the leg muscles.

Now either repeat this move on the left leg or continue on to Leg Lifts to the Side on a Mat. ▪

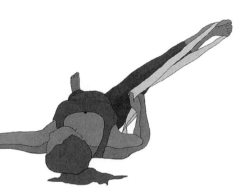

⦂ LEG LIFTS TO THE SIDE ON A MAT: After raising your leg as described in Leg Lifts, keep the right leg extended, hold both ends of the belt with just the right hand, and float the right leg over to the right. You can counterbalance by bringing the left arm and the head to the left.

Rest in this position, breathing into the right inner thigh and hip joint.

When you are ready, hold the belt in the left hand and bring the right leg as far as you can to the left, creating a stretch to the outside of the right hip and leg. Counterbalance by bringing the right arm and head to the right.

To finish this series, again hold the ends of the belt in each hand, lift the leg back to center, and reach your heel to the ceiling and then float it down to the floor. Roll both legs from side to side. Close your eyes and notice: does your right leg feel longer? Does it sink further toward the earth?

When you are ready, do the whole sequence beginning with regular Leg Lifts on the left side.

When you are finished, please rest and breathe into the effects through the whole lower body. ▪

⋮ LEGS LIFTS ON A CHAIR: This stretch is similar to the preceding Leg Lifts done on the mat.

Sit on a chair with your knees bent, feet on the floor, seat bones well anchored, belly muscles engaged, spine erect.

Put a belt around the ball of your right foot and hold the ends of the belt with each hand.

Lift the right leg toward the ceiling as straight and as high as you can. Keep your shoulders rolled back and down, away from your ears.

Position the right leg so that you can keep the right foot flexed and the right knee straight. Breathe along the back of

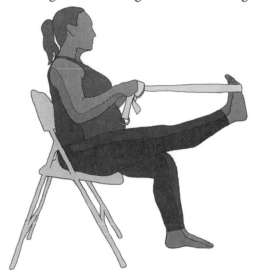

the right leg, extending the Achilles tendon, calf, and hamstring muscles.

Hold the belt in a way that allows the arms and shoulders to remain relaxed. This keeps the emphasis on stretching the leg muscles.

Now either repeat this move with the opposite leg or move on to Leg Lifts to the Side on a Chair. ∎

⦂ Leg Lifts to the Side on a Chair:

Just as with the mat variation, this pose begins with the right leg extended according to the instructions in Leg Lifts on a Chair.

Hold both ends of the belt with just the right hand.

Bring the right leg as far as possible to the right, counterbalancing by bringing the left arm and the head to the left.

Rest in the pose and breathe into the right inner thigh and hip joint.

When you are ready, hold the belt in the left hand and bring the right leg as far as you can to the left, creating a stretch to the outside of the right hip and leg. Again, you can counterbalance by extending your right arm and turning your head to the right.

To finish this series, again hold the ends of the belt in each hand and lift the right leg back to center. First reach your heel to the ceiling and then float it down to the floor. Roll both legs from side to side.

Come back to Seated Mountain Pose (page 7). Close your eyes and notice: Does your right leg feel longer or more alive?

When you are ready, do the whole sequence on the left side, beginning with Leg Lifts on a Chair.

When you're finished, please rest and breathe into the effects through the whole lower body. ∎

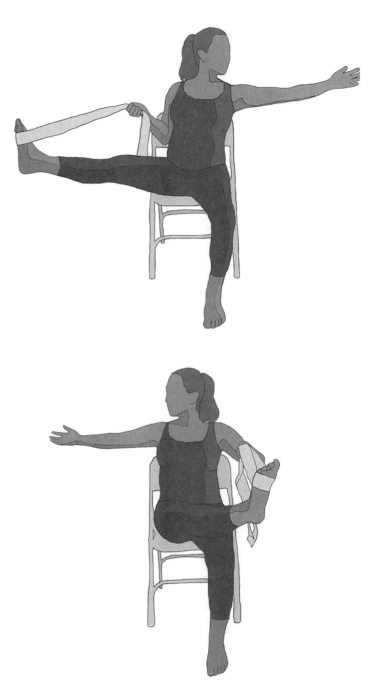

⦂ HALF FORWARD BEND ON A MAT: The benefits of this forward bend are similar to the Leg Lifts with an additional stretch along all the muscles of the back. If you find the pose challenging, you can lift the hips with a cushion or folded blanket. If you think that this form of forward bending is still too challenging for your body, remember that you do get a similar stretch through your legs with the basic Leg Lifts and you can stick with that for the time being.

When you are ready, please sit on a yoga mat in Stick Pose (pages 80–81). Lengthen your spine and legs, with the flesh of the buttocks pulled back to the wall behind you, heels pressing to the wall in front of you and the back of the knees pressing down toward the floor. Keeping your feet flexed will enhance the stretch along the backs of your legs.

Bending your left knee to the left, bring the sole of the left foot to the inner right thigh (or further down the leg if that is more comfortable).

Place a belt around the ball of your flexed right foot. Come into a forward bend, hinging forward from your hip joints, chest toward right thigh. Please keep your head in line with your spine.

If the left knee does not touch the mat, you may want to place a cushion or folded towel under it.

Find the edge of your stretch, breathing along your spine and the back of your right leg: hamstring muscles, back of the knee, calf muscle, and Achilles tendon.

Allowing the left knee to melt down, breathe into the stretch through the left hip joint.

When you are ready, release your legs, shake them out, and then repeat the Half Forward Bend on the other side. ◾

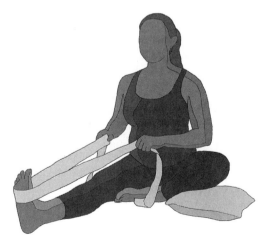

⁞ Full Forward Bend on a Mat: Again, starting from Stick Pose, hold the ends of the belt in each hand with the belt around the balls of both feet. Flex your feet and roll your shoulders up, back, and down.

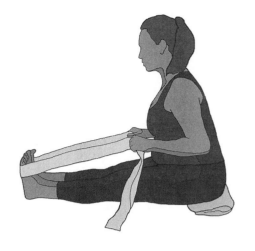

Contracting the belly muscles and lifting the breastbone to the ceiling, begin hinging forward from your hip joints, chest toward thighs, head in line with the spine. Please keep the back and the legs long and only come as far forward as you can while maintaining that length.

Inhaling, continue to open your chest and lengthen your spine; exhaling, lengthen further forward over your legs. Hold the pose for at least five deep breaths.

A variation of Full Forward Bend can be done with a bolster between the legs. Instead of holding a belt, try holding the sides of the bolster, walking your hands forward, and melting your upper body onto the bolster.

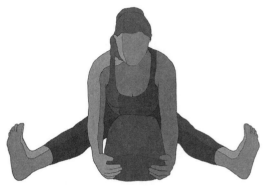

If the backs of your legs or your back muscles are not flexible, trying adding on bolsters (or cushions, pillows, or towels) so that you can rest your head, cheek to the side, and receive more of a passive stretch.

Please keep your feet flexed, backs of the legs long, and your head in line with your spine as much as possible. This pose can be very relaxing. You may want to rest in it for three to five minutes.

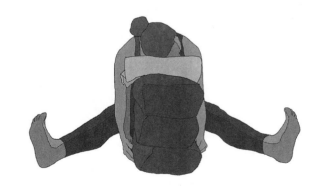

When you are ready to come out of the pose, move the bolster to the side, bring your hands to the floor on either side of your body and roll onto your back, one vertebra at a time. If you feel any discomfort in your lower back, hug your knees to your chest and rock from side to side. Take time to rest and breathe into the effects, allowing the muscles of the back and legs to sink down toward the earth. ∎

⦂ HALF FORWARD BEND ON TWO CHAIRS: For folks who prefer stretching on a chair instead of on a yoga mat, the Half and Full Forward Bends are done much the same way on a chair as on the mat. Both versions offer, in addition to the leg stretch given in Leg Lifts, a wonderful stretch for all the muscles of the back. If you find the pose challenging, you can lift the hips with a folded blanket or choose to stick with the basic Leg Lifts.

Sit in one chair and have another chair facing you. The distance between the two chairs will depend on your leg length and flexibility. For this pose it is best to use a chair without arms.

Bring both legs onto the facing chair and sit in your best version of Stick Pose (pages 80–81).

Lengthen your spine and legs, with the flesh of the buttocks pulled back to the wall behind you, heels pressed to the wall in front of you, and the backs of the knees pressed down toward the chair. Keeping your feet flexed will enhance the stretch along the backs of your legs.

Bending your left knee to the left, bring the sole of the left foot to the inner right thigh (or further down the leg if that is more comfortable).

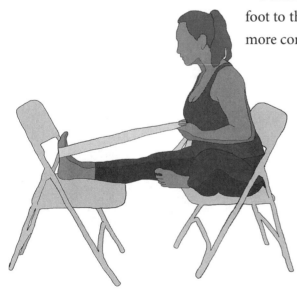

Place a belt around the ball of your flexed right foot. Come into a forward bend, hinging forward from your hip joints with your chest toward your right thigh. Please keep your head in line with your spine.

If the left knee does not touch the chair, you may want to place a cushion or folded towel under it.

Find the edge of your stretch, breathing along your spine and the back of your right leg: hamstring muscles, back of the knee, calf muscle, and Achilles tendon.

Allowing the left knee to melt down, breathe into the stretch through the left hip joint.

When you are ready, release your legs, shake them out, and repeat Half Forward Bend on the other side. ■

⁞ Full Forward Bend on Two Chairs: Start by sitting on a chair in Stick Pose with both legs stretched to the chair in front of you.

Hold the ends of the belt in each hand with the belt around the balls of both feet.

Flex your feet and roll your shoulders up, back, and down.

Contracting the belly muscles and lifting the breastbone to the ceiling, begin hinging forward from your hip joints, chest toward thighs, head in line with spine. Please keep the back and the legs long and only come as far forward as you can while maintaining that length.

Inhaling, continue to open your chest and lengthen your spine; exhaling, lengthen further forward over your legs. Hold the pose for at least five deep breaths.

When you feel finished, come back to Seated Mountain Pose (page 7). Take time to rest and breathe into the effects, allowing the muscles of the back and legs to relax completely. ■

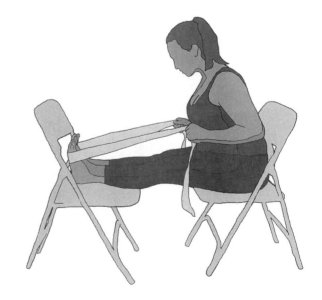

⁚ COBBLER POSE: This pose offers a gentle stretch to the hip, knee, and ankle joints and a wonderful preparation for any cross-legged sitting position. Each of the Cobbler Poses can be done on a mat or on a chair with another chair facing.

Start by sitting tall with the soles of your feet touching.

Engage the muscles of your belly, lift your spine, open your chest, and drop your shoulders away from your ears. Bring your heels toward your groin and melt your knees toward the earth.

Place your hands on your inner thighs with a slight downward pressure and then hold your feet with your hands or a belt.

If there is discomfort in your knee or hip joints, you can place cushions or folded towels under your knees or thighs.

If Cobbler Pose rounds your back, place a folded blanket or towel under your buttocks. This should shift the position of your pelvis and allow you to sit taller.

Continue to lift your spine and drop your knees. ■

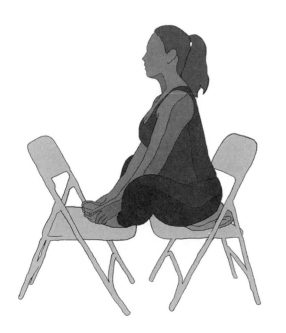
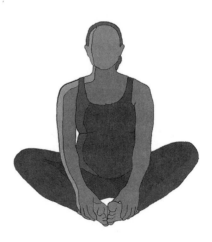

⁞ EXTENDED COBBLER POSE: This pose is a continuation of the preceding pose, adding a lovely stretch through the spine.

Keeping your knees down, lift your arms up to the ceiling; in doing so, further lengthen the spine.

Maintaining this length, fold from the hip joints, reaching your arms toward your legs, the floor, or the chair in front of you.

When you are ready to move on, release your torso and arms up and then float your arms down to the chair or floor. Extend your legs and shake them out. Please continue to sit tall and imagine that you can breathe into your feet, ankles, knees, and hips, noticing the effects of all the lower body stretches we have done. ▪

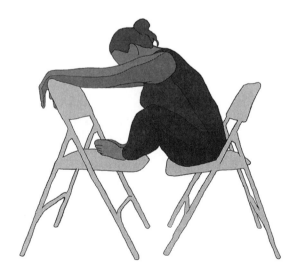

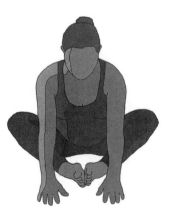

Standing Poses

*Y*OGA POSES done from a standing position are great for releasing unhappy backs, knees, and hips and for waking up a sleepy meditator. For folks with injuries or serious misalignment of the knees, hips, or spine, it is good to be aware that the following poses can strengthen needed muscles but can also sometimes exacerbate problems. It's important to do the poses with correct alignment and to back off of any pose that feels uncomfortable. If you need more guidance, please consult your healthcare provider or a certified yoga instructor to help find healthy modifications of the poses. If balance or leg strength is of concern, try using the wall or a very stable chair for support. For safety and comfort, it is wise to do all standing poses on a flat, nonslippery surface. (Wood floor is preferable to carpeting; yoga mat is preferable to bare floor.) There are seated versions of the poses offered in the next chapter for those who need a gentler, supported practice.

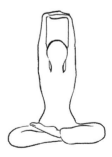

: **STANDING MOUNTAIN POSE:** A person in Standing Mountain Pose does not look like he or she is doing much more than standing tall. However, it actually takes quite a bit of strength, stamina, and loving attention to do Standing Mountain Pose properly. Establishing alignment while standing can translate into a much stronger seated posture for meditation. The exacting attention to each part of the body is in itself a wonderful meditation.

When you are first starting to work with this pose, you may want to periodically look down at your feet and knees and occasionally look in a mirror to check that you are in alignment. After you have done this enough times or perhaps worked with an instructor who has given you feedback, you will have a good sense of what means to stand like a mountain. Below are some simple guidelines.

Start by standing with your feet parallel, pointing straight ahead and just under your hip joints. For most people, your feet should be one to two fist widths apart.

Please make sure you are equally balanced on the four corners of each foot and between your two feet. Try rolling your feet side to side, in and out, forward and backward until you find balance.

Lift your toes, become aware of the resulting lift through your arches, and then bring the toes down, making sure they are well spread.

Imagine sending roots from your feet into the earth and then, from deep in the earth, imagine energy rising up through your feet, up through your legs. Engage the muscles of your lower legs, pulling the muscles in toward the bone. At the same time, tighten the quadriceps muscles (at the front of the thighs), which will in turn lift the kneecaps. Knees should be straight but not locked.

Engaging the quadriceps muscles will naturally align the pelvis, dropping the tailbone toward the earth and lifting the pubic bone toward the sky. (If you stand sideways to a mirror as you do this movement, you will see your pelvis shift and the curve at the lower back flatten a bit. If you stand facing the mirror, hopefully you will see that your hipbones are on the same plane, facing forward like two perfectly aligned headlights.)

This alignment of the pelvis helps make more space between the hip bones and the bottom of the ribs, which in turn allows us to widen the chest and breathe more fully.

We can enhance this expansion of the chest by rolling the shoulders up to the ears, back to the wall behind us, and then down toward the waist. As the shoulders rotate, allow the arms and hands to very naturally follow, with palms opening to the wall in front.

At the same time, invite alignment through the whole upper body by lengthening the spine from its base, up and out through the top of the head, while keeping the chin parallel to the earth.

Take time to breathe fully, enjoying the length and strength of your body. I think that one of the best times to do Standing Mountain Pose is when we find ourselves waiting in any very long line. Instead of being angry at the person at the front of the line (who we are sure has too many groceries or too many questions), we can pay attention to our posture and notice the story our body relays. We may notice that when we are in a rush, we may literally lean forward into the future; when we are impatient, we shift our weight from one side to the other as our mind shifts from one thing to another; when we are sad, our chest may cave in; when we are angry, our jaw may jut out. When we use that time to stand like a mountain, we can notice our inner strength, stamina, and patience, as well as the joy of being in the present moment. ■

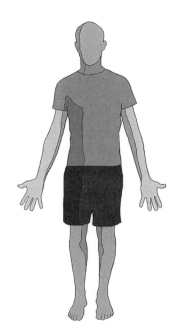

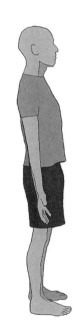

⦂ STANDING CRESCENT MOON SERIES: Standing Crescent Moon poses offer a continuation of Standing Mountain Pose with a wonderful stretch for the sides, front, and back of the body.

Rooted and aligned in Standing Mountain Pose, lift the arms overhead, either keeping the arms parallel with palms facing or clasping the hands and lifting the index fingers to the sky. As always, please honor the shoulder joints by finding a modification of this arm position as needed.

By pressing the feet and lifting the arms, maintain alignment and "grow" your body longer. This position is known as Standing Crescent Arms Up. Pressing the left foot even more strongly toward the earth, reach the arms and torso to the right, index fingers reaching for the place where ceiling and wall meet.

Breathe along the whole left side, from the left outer heel up

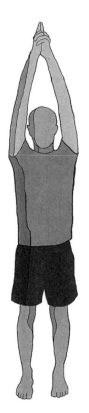 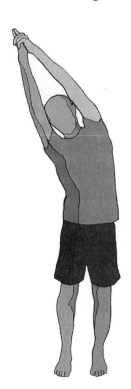 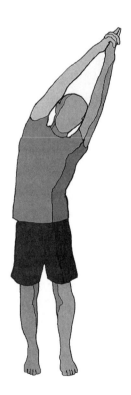

through the fingertips, expanding the left ribs on each inhalation. Please hold this pose for at least three deep breaths.

Again come back to Standing Crescent Arms Up, feet rooted to the earth and fingertips reaching to the ceiling. Apply the same stretch to the other side.

When you are ready, come back to Standing Crescent Arms Up. On an inhalation, lift your chest to the ceiling and reach your arms toward the wall behind you. Firm in your stance, press your hips forward, taking three deep breaths. This gentle stretch is the Crescent Backward Bend.

On an exhalation, swing your upper body forward, bending from your hip joints (not your waist), keeping your spine as long as you can for as long as you can. Engage the quadriceps muscles and lift the kneecaps. Pull in the abdominal muscles and reach the arms out parallel to the floor. This creates a powerful forward fold known as a Jack Knife.

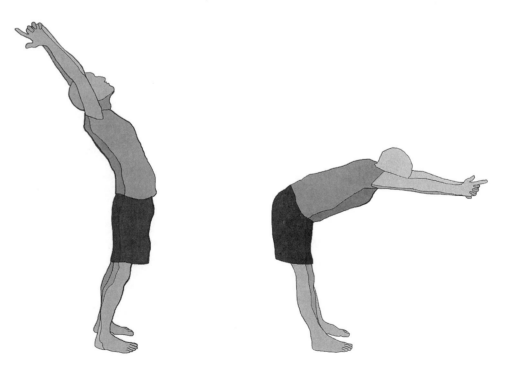

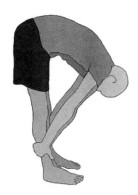

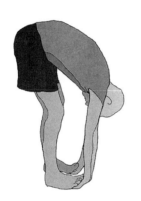

Please hold this for three breaths and then take the stretch into the deepest forward bend possible. If you can, touch your toes or the floor. You may feel more comfortable holding the backs of your legs, helping to invite the chest toward the front of the thighs. Please do not sacrifice the alignment of the spine and legs in an effort to stretch further than is appropriate for your body.

Hold your forward bend for three deep breaths and then, bending the knees as much as you need, place your palms, facing up, under the balls of your feet. From this somewhat awkward position, attempt to straighten your knees as much as possible for a strong hamstring stretch.

Release, when you are ready, back to the Jack Knife pose, then back to the Crescent Backward Bend, and back to Standing Crescent Arms Up. Slowly float your arms down to your sides. Spend three more delicious deep breaths in this fully aligned Mountain Pose, taking notice of the effects on your spine and the sides of your body, as well as any other resulting sensations. ▪

: **STANDING WARRIOR ONE:** Warrior poses, as their name implies, can bring strength, stamina, and courage to our practice. They also bring flexibility to the hips and groin area, a stretch for shoulders and arms, and relief for a tight upper back or neck.

As with most standing poses, Standing Warrior One (a front-facing variation of the pose) starts with a firm Standing Mountain Pose, arms at the sides, shoulders rolled back and down, feet rooted.

Keeping the right foot facing forward, step the left foot back three to four feet, depending on your leg length, hip flexibility, and comfort in the pose. As much as possible, have your feet, hips, and shoulders facing front. The left foot may have to turn slightly to the left for stability.

Rerooting yourself through your feet and pressing the left heel strongly into the ground, bend the right knee until it is just over the right ankle. It is important to keep the knee bent at a ninety-degree angle over the ankle and in line with the middle right toe. This helps keep all the bones of the leg in alignment.

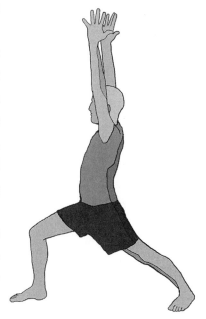

Keeping the back leg straight, imagine squeezing a beach ball between the thighs, while lengthening the spine and breathing fully into your Warrior chest.

Lifting the arms overhead can further open the chest. Palms can be facing each other or fingers interlaced with index fingers up. The lower body anchors to the earth and upper body reaches to the sky.

Hold this position while practicing either Three-Part Deep Breathing (pages 16–17) or Rapid Energizing Breathing (pages 18–19).

Please come out when you are ready. Rest in Standing Mountain Pose, conscious of your posture and breath, and then repeat the pose on the other side.

When you are finished, please take time to notice the power this pose can bring you and your capacity to come back to center, both physically and mentally. Finish with slow, deep breathing, again resting in Standing Mountain Pose. ■

⁚ STANDING WARRIOR TWO: This pose, also known as Side-Facing Warrior Pose, is similar to Standing Warrior One, but it emphasizes a stretch and strengthening of the arms and a slightly different opening for the hip joints.

Starting again from a rooted Standing Mountain Pose, keeping your right foot facing forward, bring your left foot three to four feet back with the left toes turned to about sixty degrees to the left. Please align the feet so that the right heel makes an imaginary line under the left arch.

Bring your hands to your hips and turn your hips and upper torso to the left.

Lift your arms to the ceiling, lengthening your spine.

Drop your tailbone and lift your pubic bone in order to align the pelvis.

Bring your arms out to the sides, parallel to the floor, palms down and just once roll your shoulders up, back, and down.

Turn your head to the right, bend your right knee directly over your right ankle, in line with your middle right toe. Ideally the thigh is parallel to the floor and the shinbone perpendicular to the floor. Again squeeze the inner thighs toward each other, root the feet, lengthen the spine, and stretch the arms away from each other, out through the fingertips.

Gazing past the right fingertips can enhance the sense of horizontal stretching.

Keep your spine perpendicular to the floor. Keep your breath full and deep. Imagine breathing from the base of your spine up through each of the vertebrae, out through the top of your head.

Imagine inhaling into your Warrior chest and, with each exhalation, sending power out through your arms, out through each of your fingertips, down through your legs, and through the bottom of your feet into the earth.

When you are ready to release, straighten your right knee, lift your arms to the ceiling, turn your torso to the right and step back into Standing Mountain Pose with arms floating down to the sides. Please take time to notice the effects of the pose.

Repeat Standing Warrior Two on the other side, starting again from a rooted Mountain Pose. When you are finished, take time to notice the effect of the pose on your posture, breath, and stamina. ■

⁞ STANDING TRIANGLE POSE: Standing Triangle Pose can give us additional stretching for the spine, shoulder and hip joints, and the sides of the body. It can also give a gentle massage to the internal organs. If you like using a yoga block (or a comparable prop) for support in this pose, make sure you have it near you as you move into the pose.

Starting from Standing Mountain Pose, step the left foot back three to four feet.

Keeping the right foot pointing to the right, turn your left toes about sixty degrees to the left. Please align the feet so that the right heel makes an imaginary line under the left arch.

Put your hands on your hips and turn them to the left any amount you can. Please make sure that your feet and legs feel stable and balanced, your shoulders are rolled back and down, and your spine and neck are long.

For this pose, both knees stay straight but not locked.

The spine starts perpendicular to the earth, with the tailbone down and pubic bone up, maintaining alignment of the pelvis.

Lift your arms out to the sides, parallel to the earth, palms down. Engage the muscles of your arms as you reach them away from each other. Pause and breathe, rooting through the feet, lengthening through the spine.

Shift your hips to the left and lean your torso to the right, bending from the hip joints. Becoming like a windmill, reach

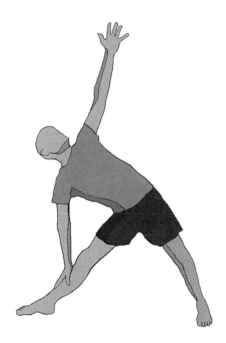

your right arm down to your right leg, to the floor or to a yoga block, placed on the right side of your right foot. Send your left arm up to the sky.

As you move more deeply into the pose, do not sacrifice the length and alignment of your spine in an effort to reach closer to the floor. It is often suggested that Standing Triangle Pose be done as if between two sheets of glass, spine parallel to the floor, arms making one long straight line.

Once you have found a position that feels strong and grounded, try pressing your right hip toward the wall in front of you and your left hip to the wall behind, lifting your chest toward the sky.

If you can comfortably, lengthen your spine and neck and turn your head to look at your top (left) thumb.

Breathe deeply into the pose and each of the affected parts of the body. Imagine making more space in the shoulders, hips, and lungs, strengthening legs and feet, and lengthening spine and arms.

When you are ready, release back into Standing Mountain Pose. Pause and breathe into the effects through your body.

Repeat Standing Triangle Pose on the other side.

When you feel finished, release back into Standing Mountain Pose. Take time to notice the effects on your legs and feet, hips, spine, and arms. Notice your breathing, your heart rate, and your ability to come back to center, rooted and tall. ■

STANDING FORWARD BEND: This form of forward bend offers a wonderful stretch for the hamstring muscles and can be profoundly relaxing for the digestive and nervous systems. It reverses the effect of gravity, bringing fresh blood to the brain and resting all the back muscles that work so hard to keep us erect. Just a short time in a Standing Forward Bend can refresh the body and the mind. If you have any physical conditions that prevent you from putting your head lower than your heart, please skip this pose.

Standing in Mountain Pose, maintaining the alignment of every part of your body, inhale and stretch your arms to the ceiling, imagining your spine growing longer.

As much as you reach up through your spine and arms, equally root down through your feet.

Continuing this lengthening and grounding, bring your hands to your hips and begin to fold forward from your hip joints (not from your waist).

Keeping the legs and spine as straight as you can, walk your hands down the back of your legs, massaging the muscles as you reach toward the floor. Stretch as far as you can. This may bring your hands as far as the back of the thighs, knees, calves, or heels. Do not sacrifice the length of your spine or legs in order to stretch further. Find the stretch that works and breathe into that.

Pulling your belly muscles in, send your hips toward the ceiling, the top of your head toward the floor, and your chest toward the front of your thighs.

If this stretch bothers your lower back, try bending your knees a bit. Otherwise, keep your knees straight but not locked.

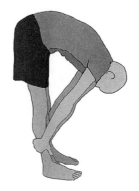

With at least three long deep breaths, stretch from your heels to your hip bones and from the base of your spine down through the top of your head.

In this position, gravity is naturally lengthening the muscles of your neck. If you would like to enhance this stretch, try shaking your head "yes" and then "no" for several rounds.

When you are ready to come out, bring your hands back to

your hips and, keeping your belly muscles engaged, slowly lift back to a rooted Mountain Pose, head coming up last. Rest your arms to your sides and breathe into the results. ■

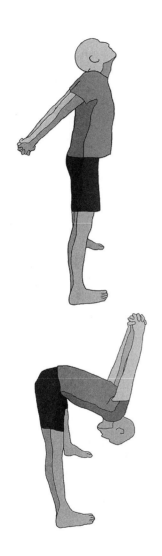

: **Standing Yoga Mudra:** In addition to bringing circulation into your shoulders and bringing increased blood flow to your spine and upper body, this pose also provides a wonderful hamstring stretch. Yoga mudra translates to mean "seal of yoga," which I was taught refers to its power to manifest one of the highest goals of yoga: melding the heart and brain.

Bring your legs 3 to 4.5 feet apart, with toes slightly facing in toward each other.

Clasp your hands behind your back. If this bothers your shoulders, hold a yoga belt (or a sock or whatever is available) between your hands.

On an inhalation, lift your chin to the ceiling and your arms as high as you can, creating a shoulder blade squeeze.

On an exhalation, bring the top of your head toward the earth and lift your clasped hands, any amount you can, toward the sky. As you pull your belly muscles in, you may be able to lift your hips even higher. If you have any physical conditions that prevent you from putting your head lower than your heart, please modify or skip this part of the pose.

Remain in this forward bend for as long as it is comfortable. Come out slowly by lifting your torso with your belly muscles engaged, continuing to lift your arms behind you, as high as you can for as long as you can.

Once you're standing upright, maintain the lift through your arms and lift your chin and chest to the ceiling. Briefly squeeze your shoulder blades together, gently arching your back.

Come back to Standing Mountain Pose. Shake your hands,

arms, and shoulders to release any residual tension. Rest your arms to the sides, taking time to breathe fully into the effects of the pose. ■

: **CAT/COW STRETCHING:** This is the same series presented on pages 50–51. I offer it here again because it is part of the Sun Salutation Series that follows in this chapter.

Start in Table Pose: on your hands and knees with your hands directly under your shoulders, your knees directly under your hips, and your back flat. You may want to provide extra padding under your knees with an extra yoga mat or blanket.

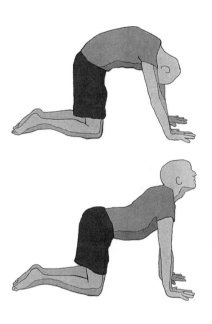

Begin with Cat Pose: on an exhalation, bring your forehead and pubic bone toward each other, rounding your back to the ceiling, like a scared cat.

Then move into Cow Pose: on an inhalation, lift your head and tailbone to the ceiling, with your spine sunk down toward the earth like a cow's spine.

Flow between these two spinal movements, guided by the breath, continuing to inhale into the Cow Pose and to exhale into the Cat Pose, allowing the spine to become quite fluid, forward and back. ■

: **DOWNWARD-FACING DOG:** This pose is often referred to as "yoga's multi-vitamin," because so many benefits are received in one simple stretch. It can strengthen and stretch shoulders, arms, hands, wrists, the whole back, hips, and legs, especially the muscles along the back of the legs: the hamstring and calf muscles, as well as the Achilles tendons. It can relax the nervous, cardiovascular, and digestive systems and bring fresh blood to the brain. The list of benefits goes on and on. And most importantly for the purposes of this book, a very short time in Downward-Facing Dog will help a tired meditator relax, release, and rejuvenate body and practice.

Prepare for Downward-Facing Dog by moving into a series of Cat/Cow Stretches. Finish with a Cow Pose.

Turn your toes under, plant your feet, and begin to straighten your knees any amount you can, sending the hips to the ceiling and the top of the head toward the floor.

Please keep the shoulders blades pressed toward each other, belly muscles engaged, and the spine long.

You may want to experiment with straightening one knee and bending the other to get a stretch along the back of one leg and then the other.

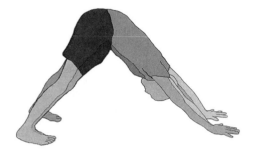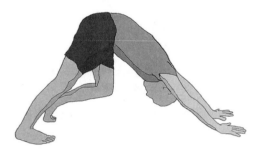

Feel free to bend both knees a bit if that is what makes holding the pose possible for you.

If you can, maintain Downward-Facing Dog with the spine long, both legs straight, both heels toward the floor. Hold the pose for at least three long deep breaths.

When you are ready to come out, walk your hands first to your feet and then up to your hips, rising slowly back into Standing Mountain Pose. Check your alignment and your capacity to again root in toward the earth. Take time to notice your breath, heart rate, and the particular benefits you have received from Downward-Facing Dog. ■

⁚ Standing Sun Salutation Series: This series offers a wonderful warm-up, including forward and backward bending poses, stretches for all the joints, and rhythmic breathing. It usually includes about twelve poses, flowing one to the next. It can be done quickly as an aerobic exercise or slowly like a dance. However it is done, this series can prepare the body for more strenuous poses or serve as a short all-encompassing exercise routine. Although there are many versions of Sun Salutations, for the purposes of this book, I will offer a simple and gentle routine, combining several poses offered previously. If you are doing the series at a slow pace, try breathing deeply throughout the sequence. For a faster version, you may want to try to inhale each time there is a backward bend, when the lungs naturally expand, and exhale on forward bends, when the lungs naturally contract. You may choose to do just one or several rounds of this series in one session.

Start in Standing Mountain Pose with your palms together at the center of your chest.

Stretch the arms overhead into a gentle backward bend. This is similar to the stretch we did in the Standing Crescent Moon Series with the chest lifted toward the ceiling and hips pressed toward the wall in front.

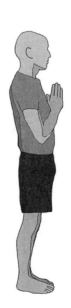
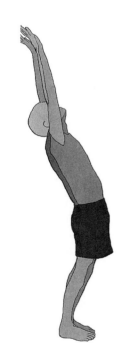

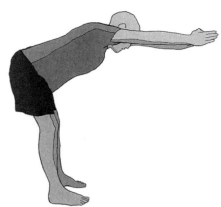

Bring your torso forward into the Jack Knife pose with your legs strong and rooted and your arms next to your ears, stretched to the wall in front.

Next, fold forward from the hip joints into any version of a Standing Forward Bend, touching your toes, the floor, your calves, the backs of your knees, or your thighs.

Bending the knees and sending the left foot back about 4 to 4.5 feet will bring you into the Runner's Lunge pose, which is wonderful for stretching the hip flexor muscles and strengthening the knees and hips.

Place the left knee on the floor for a Low Lunge.

Alternatively, you can lift the left knee for a High Lunge, which can bring a bit more weight bearing into the hip joints.

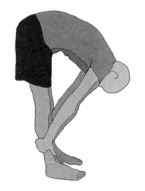 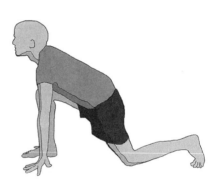

In either version of this lunge, please keep the right knee directly over the ankle, the right shin perpendicular to the floor, the chest open, and the shoulders rolled back and down. Keep the hips equidistant from the floor, both hips sinking down, almost as though they are filled with sand.

Next, swing the right foot back to meet the left, straightening the knees any amount you can, sending your hips to the ceiling and the top of your head toward the floor for Downward-Facing Dog.

You may want to bend one knee at a time, as described above.

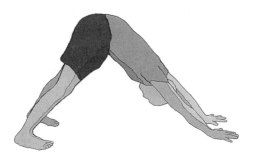 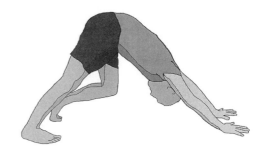

Again, feel free to bend both knees a bit if that is what makes holding the pose possible for you.

Keeping this placement of feet and hands, bring your knees to the floor and begin the Cat/Cow Stretches. On an exhalation, bring your forehead and pubic bone toward each other.

On an inhalation, lift your head and tailbone to the ceiling, allowing the spine to become quite fluid, forward and back.

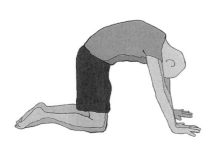 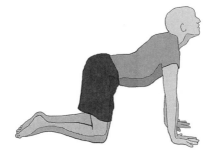

After several rounds, finish with a Cow Pose (with your tailbone and head lifted).

From here, we will run through the preceding poses again but in reverse order and on the other side of the body.

While still in Cow Pose, come on to your toes, straighten your knees any amount you can and again move into your best version of Downward-Facing Dog. Lift your hips to the ceiling and drop your heels to the floor any amount you can.

Swing the left foot forward into either the Low or High Lunge. If it is difficult to swing the left foot all the way up to be in line with the hands, then reach back behind the left ankle and invite it forward with your left hand.

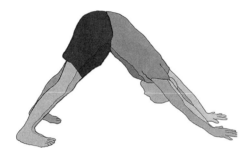 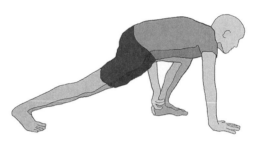

Rest in Low or High Lunge, chest open, breathing fully.

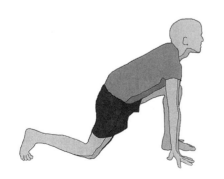 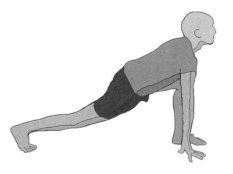

Swing your right foot forward to meet the left. Drop your head toward the floor as you raise your hips to the ceiling, coming into a Standing Forward Bend.

Reach your arms out next to or behind your ears, root through your feet, pull your belly muscles in, and lift to Standing Jack Knife Pose, spine and arms stretched forward.

Reach up to the ceiling and then back to the wall behind you, chest toward the ceiling, hips forward into a backward bend.

Finish as we started, standing tall with your palms together at the center of your chest.

Stop after one round or repeat the series as many times as you want, at a pace that suits you.

At the end of your Sun Salutation Series practice, bring awareness to the sense of circulation throughout your whole body, perhaps noticing a tingling sensation in your fingers or pulsations in other parts of your body. Please take time to notice your heart rate and breathing. Also notice your capacity to bring them back to normal with slow, deep breathing as you rest, standing tall in Standing Mountain Pose. ■

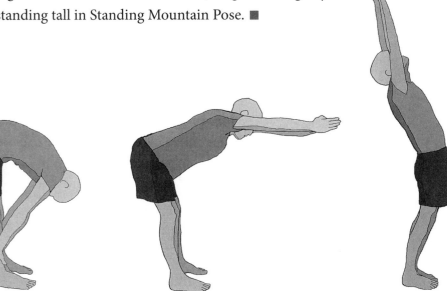

Standing Poses: Variations for Chair

: **SEATED MOUNTAIN POSE ON A CHAIR:** Mountain Pose is the basis for all seated poses and a wonderful place for realignment and rest whenever and wherever we find ourselves sitting. It takes quite a bit of strength, stamina, and loving attention to do Seated Mountain Pose in proper alignment.

Sit on a firm, comfortable chair. For stability, you may want to have the chair against a wall.

Use whatever propping you need to support you in your effort. If your feet do not touch the floor, please put a firm cushion or folded blanket under your feet. Ideally your feet are parallel, about six to eight inches apart, and should be resting solidly on whatever surface they are placed.

Please sit tall and do not lean back into the chair. If your lower back feels weak or achy, try placing a cushion under your buttocks. This can help tilt your pelvis forward, relax the muscles of your lower back, and lengthen your spine. A cushion or rolled towel at the small of your back may help you sit erect also.

Bring awareness to your feet, which should feel stable and rooted. Please make sure you are equally balanced on the four corners of each foot and between your two feet.

Lift your toes, and become aware of the resulting lift through

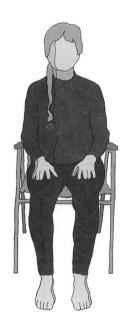

your arches. Engage the muscles of your lower legs, pulling the muscles in toward the bone. Relax the lower legs and bring the toes down, well spread. Imagine sending roots through your feet into the earth; then, from deep in the earth, imagine energy rising up through your feet, up through your legs.

Keeping your knees hip-width apart, imagine squeezing a volleyball between your knees, engaging all the muscles of the upper legs. Pull your belly muscles in, root the seat bones down, and lift up through each of the vertebrae, up through the neck and out the top of the head.

Lengthen the front of the body, making more space between the hipbones and the bottom of the ribs. This, in turn, allows one to widen the chest and breathe more fully. Enhance this expansion of the chest by rolling the shoulders up to the ears, back to the wall behind, and then down toward the waist. Ideally the shoulders are directly under the ears, and the hips are directly under the shoulders.

Keeping the chin parallel to the earth, gaze lightly to the floor or wall in front of you and rest your palms lightly on your thighs.

Please check that your hips, knees, and ankles are each bent at ninety degrees.

Take time to breathe fully, enjoying the length and strength of your body. ■

: **Crescent Moon Series on a Chair:** Crescent Moon poses offer a continuation of Seated Mountain Pose with a wonderful stretch for the sides, front, and back of the body.

Rooted and aligned in Mountain Pose, lift the arms overhead, either keeping the arms parallel to each other with palms facing or clasping the hands and lifting the index fingers to the sky. As always, please honor the shoulder joints by finding a modification of this arm position as needed.

By pressing the feet and lifting the arms, maintain alignment and "grow" your body longer. This is known as Seated Crescent Arms Up.

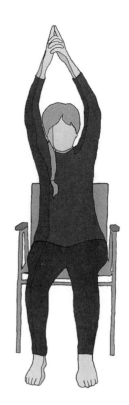

Pressing the left foot even more strongly toward the earth, reach the arms and torso to the right, index fingers reaching for the place where ceiling and wall meet. Breathe along the whole left side, from the left outer heel up to the fingertips, especially expanding the left ribs on each inhalation. Please hold this pose for at least three deep breaths.

Come back to Seated Crescent Arms Up, feet rooted to the earth, fingertips reaching to the ceiling. Apply the same stretch over to the left side. Breathe along the whole right side, from the right outer heel up to the fingertips, especially expanding the right ribs on each inhalation. Please hold for at least three deep breaths.

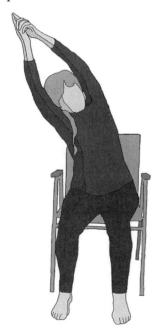

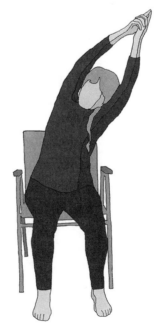

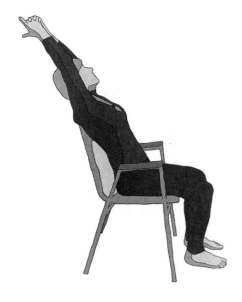

Again come back to Seated Crescent Arms Up, feet rooted to the earth and fingertips reaching for the ceiling. On an inhalation, lift your chest to the ceiling and your arms overhead to the wall behind you. Sitting firmly, press your hips forward, taking three deep breaths into this gentle backward bend.

On an exhalation, swing your torso forward, bending from your hip joints (not your waist), keeping your spine as long as you can for as long as you can. Engage the quadriceps muscles, pull in the abdominal muscles, and reach your arms out parallel to the floor. This is known as the Jack Knife.

Please hold this powerful forward fold for three breaths and then take it into the deepest full forward bend possible. (If you have any physical conditions that prevent you from putting your head lower than your heart, please skip this part of the pose.) If you can, touch your hands to your knees, shins, or toes. If you can reach the floor, place your palms on the floor on either side of your feet.

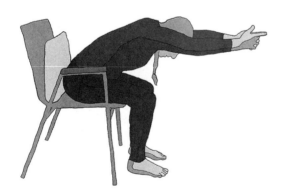

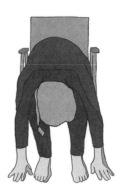

In whatever form you do this forward bend, invite the chest toward the thighs and drop the head down toward the earth, if you can do that without feeling lightheaded. Please hold this stretch for three deep breaths.

When you are ready, release back to the Jack Knife pose, then back to the back bend, and then back to Seated Crescent Arms Up. Slowly float your hands down to your thighs. Spend three more delicious deep breaths in a fully aligned Seated Mountain Pose on a Chair, taking notice of the effects on your back, spine, and the sides of your body, as well as any other resulting sensations. ■

⋮ **WARRIOR ONE ON A CHAIR:** Warrior poses, as their name implies, can bring strength, stamina, and courage to our practice. They also bring flexibility to the hips and groin area, a stretch for shoulders and arms, and relief for tight upper back and neck.

Warrior One, a front-facing version of the Warrior poses, starts with a fully aligned Seated Mountain Pose: arms at the sides, shoulders rolled back and down, feet rooted about two to three feet apart. Have the feet, hips, and shoulders facing directly forward.

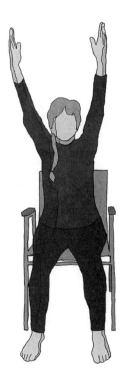

Lift the arms, palms facing each other or fingers interlaced, index fingers up.

Imagine squeezing a beach ball between the thighs, while keeping your knees apart, lengthening the spine, and breathing fully into your Warrior chest. The lower body anchors to the earth and upper body reaches to the sky.

You can nourish your body with Three-Part Deep Breathing (pages 16–17) or Rapid Energizing Breathing (pages 18–19).

When you are ready, release your hands to your thighs. Finish with slow, deep breathing, taking the time to notice the power this pose can bring you. ■

⁝ WARRIOR TWO ON A CHAIR: This warrior pose is similar to Warrior One on a Chair, but it emphasizes a different stretch and a strengthening of the arms and shoulders. It also offers a slightly different opening for the hip joints.

Start again in Seated Mountain Pose. Bring your feet two to three feet apart and turn both feet to the right.

Lift your arms to the ceiling, pull your belly muscles in, and lengthen your spine.

Bring your arms out to the sides, parallel to the floor, palms down, and, just once, roll your shoulders up, back, and down.

Turn your head to the right. Keeping the feet rooted and knees apart, squeeze the inner thighs toward each other, lengthen the spine, and stretch the arms in opposite directions, reaching out through the fingertips.

Gazing past the right fingertips can enhance the sense of horizontal stretching.

Keeping your spine perpendicular to the floor and your breath full and deep, imagine breathing from the base of your spine up through each of the vertebrae, out through the top of your head. Imagine inhaling into your Warrior chest and with each exhalation sending power out through your arms, out through each of your fingertips.

Hold the pose for at least three deep breaths.

When you are finished, come back to Seated Mountain Pose and take time to rest, allowing your breath to come back to normal.

Turn both feet to the left and please continue on to Warrior Two on the left side. Hold for at least three deep breaths.

Come out when you are ready, back to Mountain Pose, taking time to notice the echo of the pose through your body. ■

⫶ **Triangle Pose on a Chair:** Triangle Pose can give us additional stretching for the spine, shoulders, hips, and the sides of the body.

Start from Warrior Two pose, with legs two to three feet apart, arms stretched to the sides, and toes and head turned to the right.

Root the seat bones down, pull the belly muscles in, and lift the spine and neck.

Engage the muscles of your arms as you reach them in opposite directions, palms down.

Shift your hips to the left and lean your torso to the right. Becoming like a windmill, reach your right arm down toward the earth and send your left arm up to the sky. As you move more deeply into the pose, do not sacrifice the length and alignment of your spine in an effort to reach closer to the floor. Your arms should make one long straight line.

Once you have found a position that feels strong and grounded, try pressing your right hip toward the wall in front of you and your left hip toward the wall behind, lifting your chest toward the sky.

If you can comfortably, lengthen your spine and neck and then turn your head to look at your top (left) thumb.

Breathe deeply into the pose and each of the affected parts of the body; imagine making more space in the shoulders, hips, and lungs, strengthening legs and feet, lengthening arms and spine.

When you are ready, release back into Warrior Two, turning toes and head to the left. Repeat Triangle Pose to the other side.

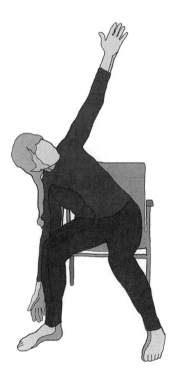

When you are ready, release back into Mountain Pose, back to center. Please take time to notice the effect of all these poses on your posture, breathing, and stamina. ■

⦂ **SEATED FORWARD BENDS ON A CHAIR:** All forward bends give a great stretch for the back and spine, a gentle massage to the digestive organs, and increased blood flow to the brain. See which of the forward bends described below work best for you.

Rooted and aligned in Seated Mountain Pose, lift the arms overhead. As always, please honor the shoulder joints by finding a modification of this arm position as needed.

By pressing the feet and lifting the arms, maintain alignment and inhale your body longer.

On an exhalation, pivot forward, bending from your hip joints (not your waist), keeping your spine as long as you can, parallel to the floor. Engage the quadriceps muscles, pull in the abdominal muscles, and reach your arms out to create the powerful Jack Knife forward fold.

Please hold this for at least three breaths.

From Jack Knife pose, move into the deepest forward bend possible.

You may be able to touch your shins or toes. If you can reach the floor, place your palms on the floor on either side of your feet.

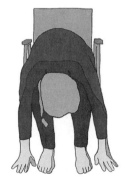

Please modify the pose to work for your body. If you get lightheaded dropping your head toward the floor, or if you have any physical conditions that prevent you from putting your head lower than your heart, it is fine to bring your hands to your thighs or knees and stretch forward instead of down.

You can also do this pose with your legs stretched out as far as they will go, feet planted, arms reaching down your legs. This will provide a somewhat stronger stretch for the lower back. Do this pose sitting at the front edge of your chair.

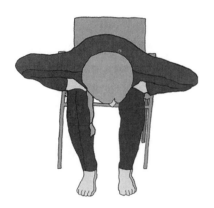 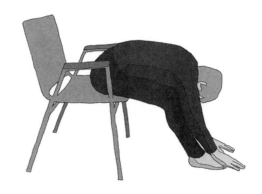

In whatever form you do forward bends, invite the chest toward the front of the thighs and keep the head in line with the spine. Please hold the pose for at least three deep breaths. When you are ready, release back to Jack Knife pose, then back up to Seated Mountain Pose. Sit tall, noticing the effect through all the muscles of your back, neck, shoulders, and arms. Notice your heart rate and breathing. Slow it all down with full, deep breathing. ■

: Yoga Mudra on a Chair: In addition to bringing circulation into your shoulders, this pose brings increased blood flow to your spine and upper body. *Yoga mudra* translates to mean

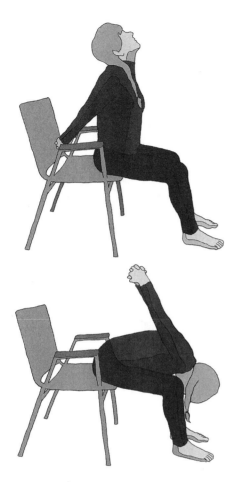

"seal of yoga," which refers to its power to manifest one of the highest goals of yoga: melding the heart and brain.

Sit firmly in Mountain Pose at the front edge of your chair with your spine long and your feet rooted about two to three feet apart. You may want to slightly turn your toes in toward each other.

Clasp your hands behind your back. If this bothers your shoulders, hold a yoga belt (or a sock or whatever is available) between your hands.

On an inhalation, lift your chin to the ceiling and your arms as high as you can, creating a shoulder blade squeeze.

On an exhalation, drop the top of your head toward the floor, lean forward from your hips, and lift your clasped hands any amount you can. Modify the pose as needed and remain in it for at least three deep breaths.

Come out slowly by engaging your belly muscles, lifting your torso, and continuing to raise your arms off your back, as high as you can for as long as you can.

Keeping your arms up, lift your chin and chest to the ceiling, briefly and gently arching your back. When you feel ready, come back to sitting tall, resting your palms on your thighs, taking time to breathe fully into the results. ∎

⁝ **Sun Salutation Series on a Chair:** This series offers a wonderful warm-up, including forward and backward bending poses, stretches for the joints, and rhythmic breathing. There are many versions of Sun Salutations. Usually it includes about twelve poses, flowing from one to the next. The poses can be done quickly, almost as an aerobic exercise, or slowly, like a dance. However it is done, this series can prepare the body for a full yoga session or serve as a short all-encompassing exercise routine. If you are doing it at a slow pace, try breathing deeply throughout the sequence. For a faster version, you may want to try to inhale each time there is a backward bend, when the lungs naturally expand, and exhale on forward bends, when the lungs naturally contract. You may choose to do just one or several rounds of this series in one session. Although traditionally this series is done from a standing position, students are often amazed by how much of a stretch, even an aerobic workout, they receive from the following chair sequence.

Start in Seated Mountain Pose, conscious of rooting through the feet and aligning through the body. On an exhalation, bring the palms together at the center of the chest.

On an inhalation, stretch the arms overhead.

On an exhalation, move forward into Jack Knife pose with your legs strong and rooted, arms next to the ears and stretched to the wall in front.

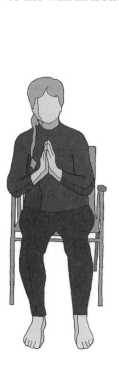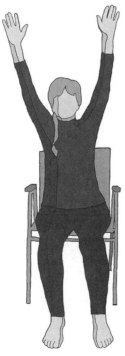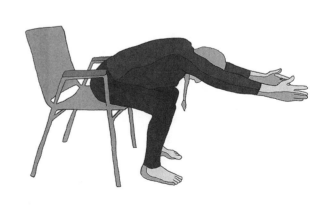

Next, fold forward from the hip joints into any version of a Seated Forward Bend, touching the knees, shins, toes, or floor.

On an inhalation, sit back up and hug your right knee toward your chest with both hands, while lifting your chin to the ceiling.

Exhaling, bring your forehead and right knee toward each other.

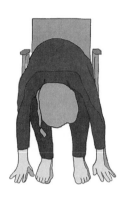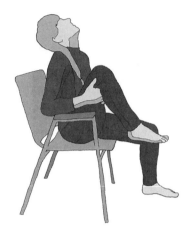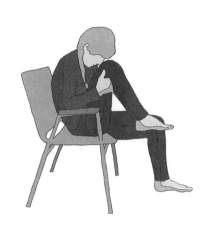

Lower the right foot to the floor as you again inhale and lift your arms.

Exhale again into the Jack Knife pose.

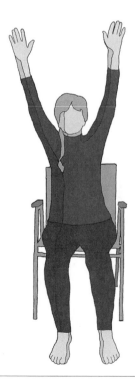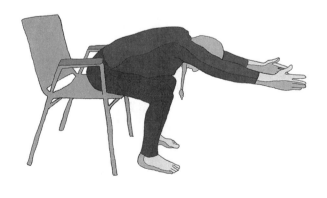

Fold from the hip joints into any version of a Seated Forward Bend.

Inhaling, hug the left knee to the chest with both hands, while lifting the chin to the ceiling.

Exhaling, bring your forehead and left knee toward each other.

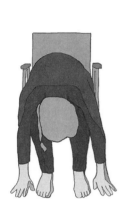 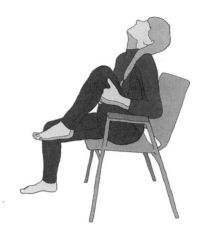 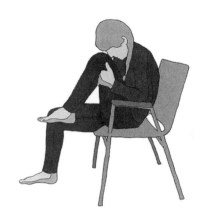

Lower the left foot to the floor as you inhale and lift your arms. Finish as you began: in Seated Mountain Pose, exhaling, bringing your palms together at the middle of your chest. This constitutes one round of Sun Salutation Series on a Chair. You can stop here or do several more continuous rounds.

Finish by enjoying some long, slow, deep breaths, noticing each part of your body that is well stretched. ■

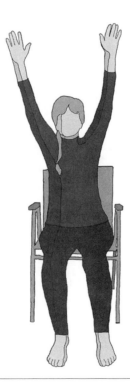

Relaxation

MOST YOGA INSTRUCTORS suggest that any series of stretches should end with at least a short time of relaxation in order to fully absorb the effects of the poses. If you spend twenty to thirty minutes stretching, spend at least three minutes relaxing at the end of your session. Even if you just spend three minutes stretching, pause at the end to be aware of each part of your body and to have some slow, deep breaths. Many people feel they can skip this aspect of yoga practice—they think that the poses are really the important part and the relaxation is just icing on the cake. But by skipping this portion of a session, much of the value of practice is lost. Conscious resting gives time for the breath and heart rate to slow; for previously held toxins to leave the body and fresh oxygen to nourish every cell; for the organs and glands, blood, and lymph systems to find equilibrium; for the entire nervous system to thoroughly rest. It is a perfect preparation for meditation.

I also suggest having a short relaxation at the beginning of each session. Doing so offers an opportunity to downshift from daily life into a slower pace that helps facilitate conscious stretching.

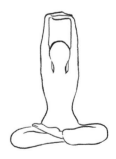

: **BODY SCAN:** This technique, if practiced before stretching, helps us pay intimate attention to exactly what kind of stretching our body needs, where we may need to be careful, where we may be ready for an extra challenge. Spending just one minute scanning through the body can transform our movements into a form of meditation.

Find a comfortable position on a mat or on a chair and bring your awareness to your feet and lower legs, around the knees, and up through the thighs. Be aware of any areas of current or old injuries, any sense of imbalance or tension. Bring this kind of awareness up through the hips, buttocks, belly, and lower back. Pay attention to the ribs and middle back, chest, and upper back. Notice where and how you feel the breath: Is it deep or shallow, coming in through the nose or mouth, filling the whole lung capacity or just the upper lungs? Is the breath flowing easily or is it constricted? Bring this inner flashlight of awareness along the spine to the neck and throat, face and scalp, and finally to the eyes. Notice any sensations around or behind the eyes. Take one long deep breath to fill each of these parts of your body and, on the exhalation, imagine the breath sweeping through you, head to toe, like a cleansing breeze. Rest with the results of this body scan, with any information you gleaned and then move, when you are ready, into your stretching session. ■

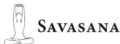 **SAVASANA**

The suggested pose for relaxation at the end of a yoga session is called *Savasana*, which translates from Sanskrit as "corpse pose"—this indicates just how deeply you are invited to rest. If you are doing Savasana lying down, you may want to place an eye pillow over the eyes. This can block light and relax the eyes, the area around and behind the eyes, the optic nerve, and the brain, resting the whole nervous system. Savasana is usually done lying on the floor, but you can also do Savasana while seated on a chair. Whichever version you choose, it is a good idea to have an extra blanket handy to cover you. We often lose body heat as we rest and our body systems slow down.

To ensure total letting go, you may want to record yourself reading the following guided relaxation. This will enable you to listen to the recording and be effortlessly led through this process of resting deeply whenever you want. If you do so, make sure to leave adequate moments of silence in the recording to let yourself fully relax into each step along the way. You may prefer to use the *Sit with Less Pain* companion CDs. (Ordering information is in the resources section at the back of this book.)

: Savasana on a Mat: Lie flat on your back with as much padding as you need to be comfortable. You may want to place a folded towel under your head and a cushion under your knees.

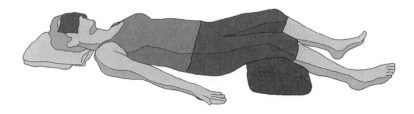

Lengthen the back of your neck with both hands, gently pulling your head toward the wall behind you. After you rest your head down to the floor, tuck the chin toward the chest to help maintain that length.

Allow your legs to rest about twelve to eighteen inches apart.

Rest your arms away from the sides of your body, palms facing the ceiling.

Make sure both the arms and both the legs are equidistant from the midline of the body—that is, one limb should not be at a different angle than the other.

Begin with a scan of the body, noticing any places of residual tension or imbalance from the right to the left and from the front to the back of the body. Notice any particular effects from the stretching you did.

Notice the flow of your breathing, the state of your mind, the quality of your attention.

Imagine any residual tension or achiness in any part of your body moving down into your right foot. On an inhalation, squeeze your right foot, and then your whole right leg, and lift them about three inches off the floor. Hold the inhalation, squeeze harder, and then on a loud exhalation, drop the leg, roll it from side to side, and allow any tension to flow out through the tips of the toes.

Do the same thing on the left side: On an inhalation, squeeze and lift the left foot and leg, hold the squeeze and the inhalation, and then on a sounding exhale, let it go. Roll both legs from side to side and allow them both to sink down and release fully.

Bring your awareness to both of your hands. Squeeze them into fists, stretch the fingers, and then tighten into fists again. On an inhalation, lift your straight arms three inches, hold, and on a sounding exhale, drop them. Roll your arms side to side and then let them go.

Lift your hips on an inhalation; on the exhalation, drop them, and roll them from side to side.

Squeeze your shoulders together in front, then behind, then

up to your ears while scrunching up your face. On the exhalation, release your face and drop your shoulders and roll them from side to side.

Stick out your tongue, lift your eyebrows, stretch your face, and on an exhalation, let your facial muscles soften.

If any other part of your body still feels tense, squeeze that part, lift it, hold it, and then release and let it melt.

Imagine relaxation spreading from the bottoms of your feet and toes, up through the tops of your feet, ankles, and calves, and around and behind your knees, upper legs, and thighs. Allow your feet and legs to feel heavy and sink toward the earth. Send the same relaxation through your fingers, hands, and arms, up to and through your shoulders. Allow your shoulders to also sink toward the earth. Bring this awareness to the base of your spine and up through each of the vertebrae, up through your neck, and up and out through the top of your head. Bring your awareness to the muscles of your lower, middle, and upper back, especially to the muscles that run along either side of the spine. Bring this sensation of relaxation to your belly muscles, ribs, and chest and to all the organs inside, each settling into just the right place.

Again become aware of the flow of your breath and of your own heartbeat. Pause here to stay awhile with the sensations of these inner rhythms.

Bring awareness to your neck and throat and jaw. Melt the muscles of your face, around and behind your ears, around your nose and cheeks, across your forehead and scalp, and especially around and behind your eyes.

Feel the support of the floor under your body and allow your body to deeply rest. Pause here for a least one minute, for longer if you want.

When you are ready to come out, do so slowly. Be aware again of your breathing and let it get deeper. Wiggle your fingers and toes; stretch your legs and arms. Stretch your whole body in any way that is pleasurable to you and then slowly roll to one side into a fetal position. Rest here for at least thirty seconds.

When you are ready, push with your top hand to help you come back up to sitting. Take time to notice the effects of this relaxation and the whole yoga session on your body and mind. Please bring the effects with you, into your sitting practice and into your life. ■

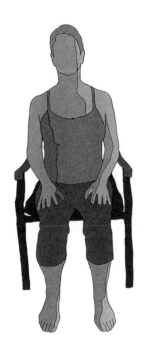

: **SAVASANA ON A CHAIR:** Please make sure your body is in alignment and supported for a complete rest.

Roll the shoulders up back and down, creating a bit of a shoulder blade squeeze, and then allow the shoulders to melt toward the earth.

Begin with a scan of the body, noticing any places of residual tension or imbalance from the right to the left and from the front to the back of the body. Notice any particular effects from the stretching you did.

Notice the flow of your breathing, the state of your mind, the quality of your attention.

Imagine any residual tension or achiness in any part of your body moving down into your right foot. On an inhalation, squeeze your right foot, and then your whole right leg, and then lift your extended leg about three inches off the floor. Hold the inhalation, squeeze harder, and then on a loud exhalation drop the leg, roll it from side to side, and allow any tension to flow out through your right toes.

Do the same thing on the left side: On an inhalation, squeeze and lift the left foot and leg, hold the squeeze and the inhalation, and then on a sounding exhale, let it go. Roll both legs from side to side and allow them both to sink down and release fully.

Bring your awareness to both of your hands. Squeeze them into fists, stretch the fingers, and then tighten into fists again. On an inhalation, lift your straight arms out to the sides and on a sounding exhale drop them. Shake your arms and then let them go.

Inhaling, tighten the muscles of your buttocks. On an exhalation, drop them, and roll them from side to side.

Squeeze your shoulders together in front, then behind, then up to your ears while scrunching up your face. On the exhalation, release your face and drop your shoulders and shake them from side to side.

Stick out your tongue, lift your eyebrows, stretch your face, and on an exhalation, let your facial muscles soften.

If any other part of your body still feels tense, squeeze that part, lift it, hold it, and then release and let it melt.

Imagine relaxation spreading from the bottoms of your feet and toes, up through the tops of your feet, ankles, and calves, and around and behind your knees, upper legs, and thighs. Allow your feet and legs to feel heavy and sink toward the earth. Send the same relaxation through your fingers, hands, and arms, up to and through your shoulders. Allow your shoulders to also sink toward the earth. Bring this awareness to the base of your spine and up through each of the vertebrae, up through your neck, and up and out through the top of your head. Bring your awareness to the muscles of your lower, middle, and upper back, especially to the muscles that run along either side of the spine. Bring this sensation of relaxation to your belly muscles, ribs, and chest and to all the organs inside, each settling into just the right place.

Again become aware of the flow of your breath and of your own heartbeat. Pause here to stay awhile with the sensations of these inner rhythms.

Bring awareness to your neck and throat and jaw. Melt the muscles of your face, around and behind your ears, around your nose and cheeks, across your forehead and scalp, and especially around and behind your eyes.

Feel the support of the chair under your body and allow your body to deeply rest. Pause here for a least one minute, for longer if you want.

When you are ready to come out, do so slowly. Be aware again of your breathing and let it get deeper. Wiggle your fingers and toes; stretch your legs and arms. Stretch your whole body in any way that is pleasurable to you. Rest here for at least thirty seconds, quietly becoming a witness to the breath flowing in and out, to the fresh energy filling the body.

Take time to notice the effects of this relaxation and the whole yoga session on your body and mind. Please bring the effects with you, into your sitting practice and into your life. ■

Suggested Sequences of Poses

CHOOSING WHICH POSES to do and when to do them will depend on your schedule, your circumstances, and your needs. In general, teachers suggest that yoga be done on an empty stomach, in a place that is quiet and tranquil, and at a time one can focus on the movements of body and breath. Traditionally, it is suggested that yoga be done at least once or twice daily, in the early morning and/or the early evening. These are naturally quiet times, before big meals, that may work well for your schedule and your daily rhythms. If, because of family or work demands, these guidelines are not appropriate for you, then do what works.

For instance, I have memories of squeezing yoga sessions into my children's nap times. I trained myself to hear their waking cries to be the same as the bell that signals the end of a sitting. I would bow, pick them up, and move on. I also have memories of sitting with a sangha that did not allow stretching during meditation retreats; yoga was seen as a serious detour from practice. I am only a little embarrassed to report that during those years, I did some great yoga stretching in the tiny bathroom next to the zendo, during walking meditation.

If your goal is just to prepare for or release from meditation, then doing the poses you most need just before or after sitting

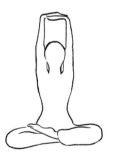

is fine. If you find that you would like to have longer yoga sessions, you may want to try one of the suggested series of poses below. I think it is most important to give yourself exactly what you need with full attention. Allow the stretching to become your practice while you are doing it—not one more thing to rush through so you can check it off your to-do list.

Allow at least three deep breaths for each pose, more if you wish. You may want to turn off your phone, tell the folks you live with that you will need some quiet time, or put up a friendly sign to request quiet. In order to settle into stretching-as-practice, it helps to start even a short yoga session with the Body Scan (page 130) and end with some version of Savasana (pages 130–36) and conscious deep breathing (any of the exercises on pages 14–17).

On the following pages, some of the illustrations are for chair poses, some are for mat poses, and some can serve for both chair and mat poses.

Five-Minute Sequence on a Mat

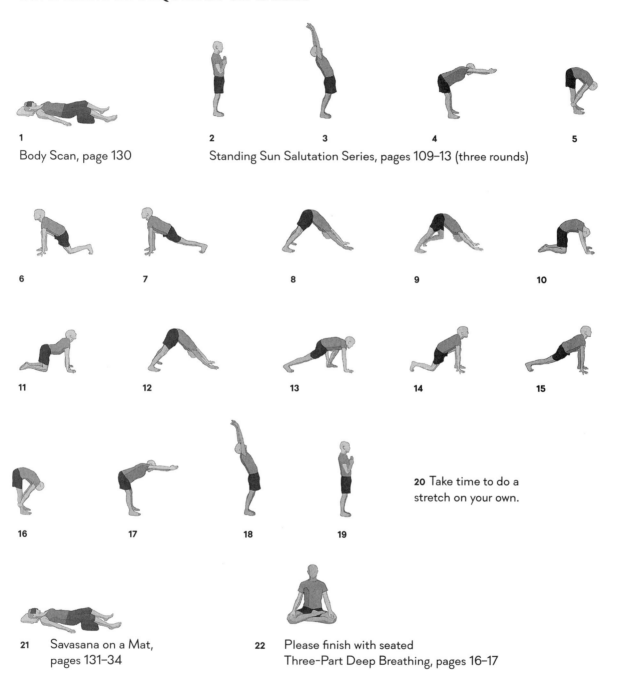

1
Body Scan, page 130

2   **3**   **4**   **5**
Standing Sun Salutation Series, pages 109–13 (three rounds)

6   **7**   **8**   **9**   **10**

11   **12**   **13**   **14**   **15**

16   **17**   **18**   **19**

20 Take time to do a stretch on your own.

21 Savasana on a Mat, pages 131–34

22 Please finish with seated Three-Part Deep Breathing, pages 16–17

FIVE-MINUTE SEQUENCE ON A CHAIR

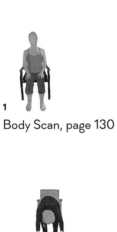

1
Body Scan, page 130

2   **3**   **4**
Sun Salutation Series on a Chair, pages 124–27 (three rounds)

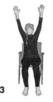

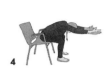

5   **6**   **7**   **8**

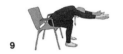

9   **10**   **11**   **12**

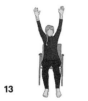

13   **14**   **15**   Take time to do a stretch on your own.

16
Savasana on a Chair,
pages 134–36

17
Please finish with seated Three-Part
Deep Breathing, pages 16–17

Relaxing Sequence on a Mat

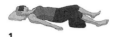

1

Body Scan, page 130

2

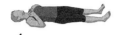

3

4

Three-Part Deep Breathing, pages 16–17

5

Alternate Nostril Breathing, page 18

6 Vertical Eye Movements, page 22 (four repetitions)
Horizontal Eye Movements, page 22 (four repetitions)
Diagonal Eye Movements, page 22 (four repetitions)
Circular Eye Movements, page 22 (four repetitions)

7

Eye Release, page 23

8

TMJ Movement and Release, page 23

9 **10**

Neck Stretches, Forward and Back, page 24 (four repetitions)

11 **12**

Neck Stretches, Side to Side, pages 24–25 (four repetitions)

13

Neck Stretches, Ear to Shoulder, pages 25–26

14 **15**

Shoulder Circles, page 26 (four forward and four back with your hands on your shoulders, and four forward and four back with your arms stretched in opposite directions)

16 **17**

Elbow/Shoulder Movements, page 27 (repeat the whole sequence four times)

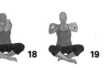

18 **19**

continues on next page

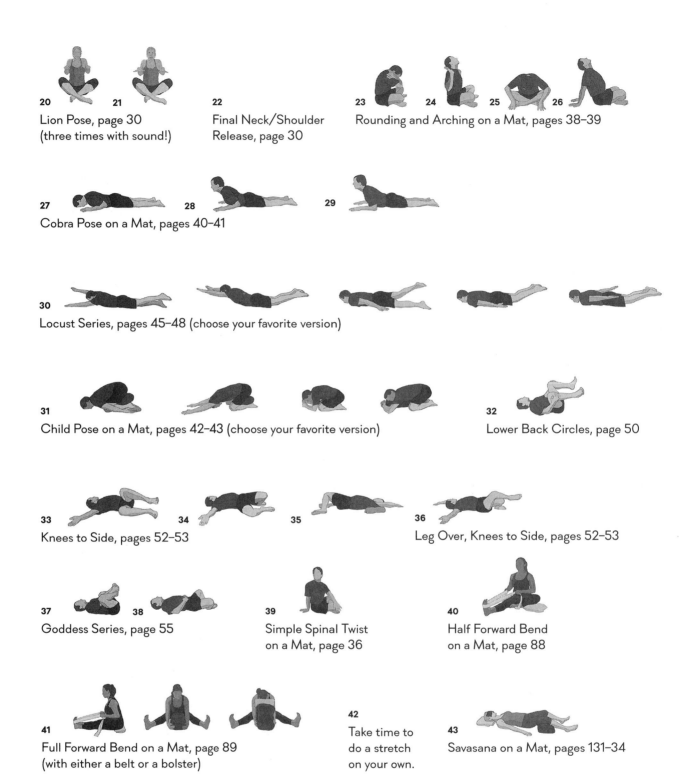

20 **21** Lion Pose, page 30 (three times with sound!)

22 Final Neck/Shoulder Release, page 30

23 **24** **25** **26** Rounding and Arching on a Mat, pages 38–39

27 **28** **29** Cobra Pose on a Mat, pages 40–41

30 Locust Series, pages 45–48 (choose your favorite version)

31 Child Pose on a Mat, pages 42–43 (choose your favorite version)

32 Lower Back Circles, page 50

33 **34** **35** Knees to Side, pages 52–53

36 Leg Over, Knees to Side, pages 52–53

37 **38** Goddess Series, page 55

39 Simple Spinal Twist on a Mat, page 36

40 Half Forward Bend on a Mat, page 88

41 Full Forward Bend on a Mat, page 89 (with either a belt or a bolster)

42 Take time to do a stretch on your own.

43 Savasana on a Mat, pages 131–34

Relaxing Sequence on a Chair

1
Body Scan, page 130

2
Three-Part Deep
Breathing, pages 16–17

3
Alternate Nostril
Breathing, page 18

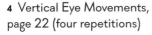

4 Vertical Eye Movements,
page 22 (four repetitions)

5 Horizontal Eye
Movements, page 22
(four repetitions)

6 Diagonal Eye
Movements, page 22
(four repetitions)

7 Circular Eye
Movements, page 22
(four repetitions)

8 Eye Release, page 23

9
TMJ Movement and
Release, page 23

10 **11**
Neck Stretches, Forward
and Back, page 24 (four
repetitions)

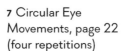

12 **13**
Neck Stretches, Side to Side,
pages 24–25 (four repetitions)

14
Neck Stretches, Ear to Shoulder,
pages 25–26 (one long stretch to
each side)

15 **16**
Shoulder Circles, page 26 (four forward and
four back with your hands on your shoulders,
and four forward and four back with your arms
stretched in opposite directions)

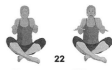

17 **18** **19** **20**
Elbow/Shoulder Movements, page 27 (repeat
the whole sequence four times)

21 **22**
Lion Pose, page 30
(three times with sound!)

23
Final Neck/Shoulder
Release, page 30

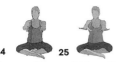

24 **25** **26** **27** **28** **29** **30**
Finger/Hand/Wrist Stretches, pages 31–33

continues on next page

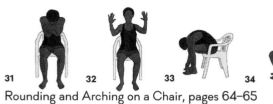

31 **32** **33** **34** **35** **36**

Rounding and Arching on a Chair, pages 64–65

Middle Back Squeeze on a Chair, pages 65–66

Seated Backward Bend on a Chair, page 69

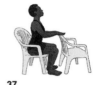
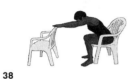

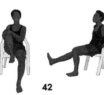

37 **38** **39** **40** **41** **42**

Cobra/Child Pose on a Chair, pages 66–67

Hip-Stretching Sequence on a Chair, pages 69–71

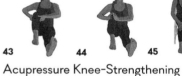
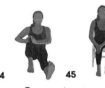

43 **44** **45** **46**

Acupressure Knee-Strengthening Exercise, pages 79–80

Chair Stick Pose, pages 80–81

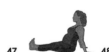
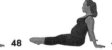
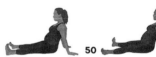

47 **48** **49** **50** **51**

Foot Stretches, pages 81–82

Half Forward Bend on Two Chairs, pages 90–91

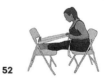

52 **53** **54** Take time to do a stretch on your own. **55**

Full Forward Bend on Two Chairs, page 91

Simple Spinal Twist on a Chair, pages 61–62 (with your knees to the side if necessary)

Savasana on a Chair, pages 134–36

Energizing Sequence on a Mat

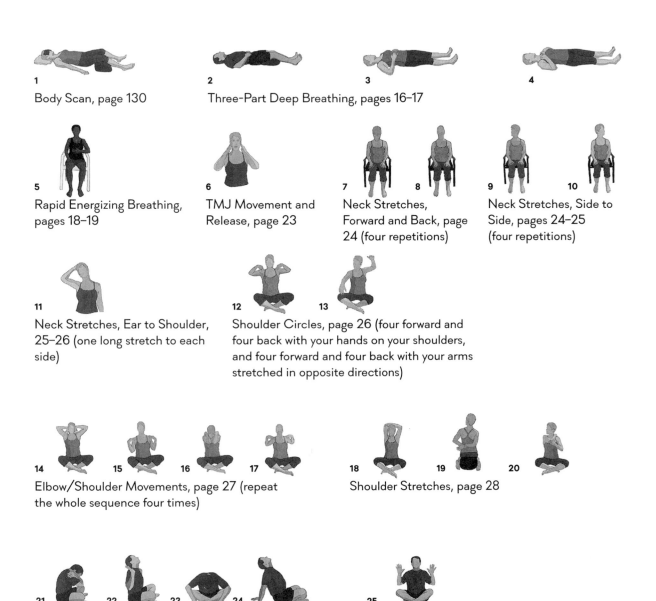

1
Body Scan, page 130

2 **3** **4**
Three-Part Deep Breathing, pages 16–17

5
Rapid Energizing Breathing, pages 18–19

6
TMJ Movement and Release, page 23

7 **8**
Neck Stretches, Forward and Back, page 24 (four repetitions)

9 **10**
Neck Stretches, Side to Side, pages 24–25 (four repetitions)

11
Neck Stretches, Ear to Shoulder, 25–26 (one long stretch to each side)

12 **13**
Shoulder Circles, page 26 (four forward and four back with your hands on your shoulders, and four forward and four back with your arms stretched in opposite directions)

14 **15** **16** **17**
Elbow/Shoulder Movements, page 27 (repeat the whole sequence four times)

18 **19** **20**
Shoulder Stretches, page 28

21 **22** **23** **24**
Rounding and Arching on a Mat, pages 38–39

25
Middle Back Squeeze on a Mat, page 39

continues on next page

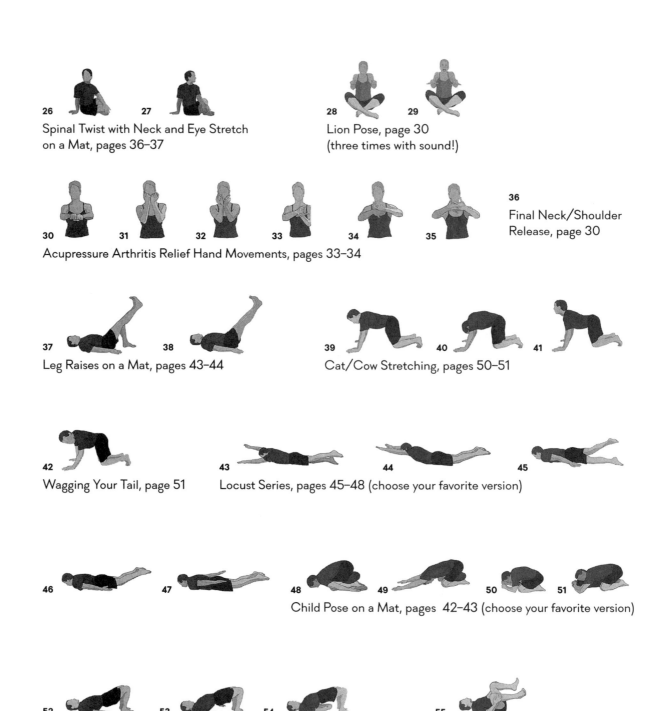

26 **27** Spinal Twist with Neck and Eye Stretch on a Mat, pages 36–37

28 **29** Lion Pose, page 30 (three times with sound!)

30 **31** **32** **33** **34** **35** Acupressure Arthritis Relief Hand Movements, pages 33–34

36 Final Neck/Shoulder Release, page 30

37 **38** Leg Raises on a Mat, pages 43–44

39 **40** **41** Cat/Cow Stretching, pages 50–51

42 Wagging Your Tail, page 51

43 **44** **45** Locust Series, pages 45–48 (choose your favorite version)

46 **47**

48 **49** **50** **51** Child Pose on a Mat, pages 42–43 (choose your favorite version)

52 **53** **54** Bridge Pose, pages 48–49 (choose your favorite version)

55 Lower Back Circles, page 50

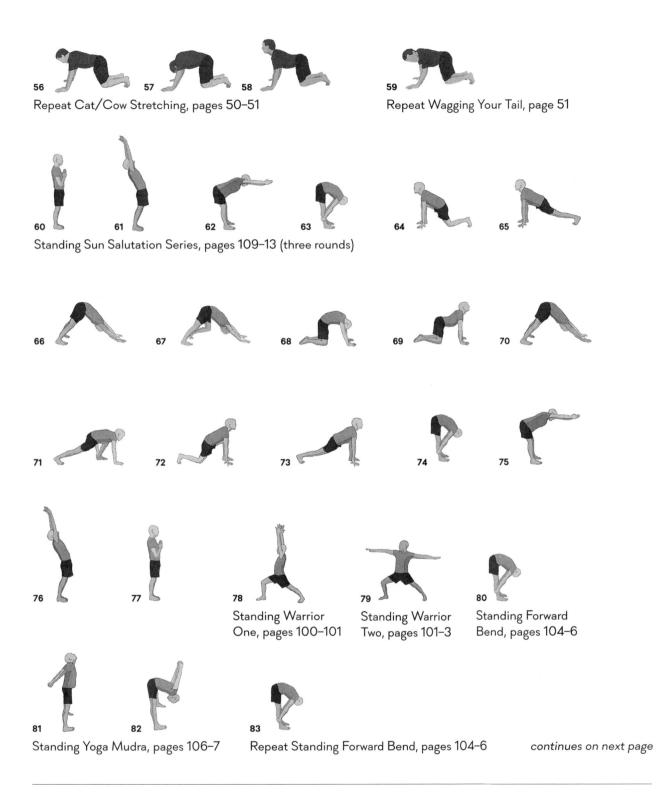

56 **57** **58**   **59**

Repeat Cat/Cow Stretching, pages 50–51   Repeat Wagging Your Tail, page 51

60 **61** **62** **63** **64** **65**

Standing Sun Salutation Series, pages 109–13 (three rounds)

66 **67** **68** **69** **70**

71 **72** **73** **74** **75**

76 **77** **78** **79** **80**

Standing Warrior One, pages 100–101

Standing Warrior Two, pages 101–3

Standing Forward Bend, pages 104–6

81 **82** **83**

Standing Yoga Mudra, pages 106–7   Repeat Standing Forward Bend, pages 104–6   *continues on next page*

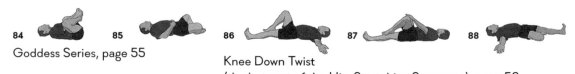

84 **85** **86** **87** **88**

Goddess Series, page 55

Knee Down Twist
(the last part of the Hip-Stretching Sequence), page 58

89 Take time to do
a stretch on your own.

90

Savasana on a Mat, pages 131–34

ENERGIZING SEQUENCE ON A CHAIR

(Two sturdy chairs are needed for this sequence)

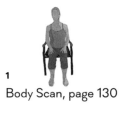   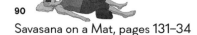

1

Body Scan, page 130

2

Three-Part Deep
Breathing, pages 16–17

3

Rapid Energizing
Breathing, pages 18–19

4

TMJ Movement and
Release, page 23

5 **6**

Neck Stretches, Forward and Back,
page 24 (four repetitions)

7 **8**

Neck Stretches, Side to Side,
pages 24–25 (four repetitions)

9

Neck Stretches, Ear to
Shoulder, pages 25–26

10 **11**

Shoulder Circles, page 26 (four forward and four back with your hands on your shoulders,
and four forward and four back with your arms stretched in opposite directions)

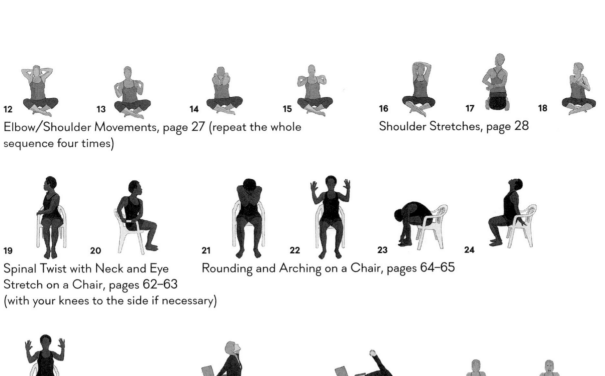

12 **13** **14** **15** **16** **17** **18**

Elbow/Shoulder Movements, page 27 (repeat the whole sequence four times)

Shoulder Stretches, page 28

19 **20** **21** **22** **23** **24**

Spinal Twist with Neck and Eye Stretch on a Chair, pages 62–63 (with your knees to the side if necessary)

Rounding and Arching on a Chair, pages 64–65

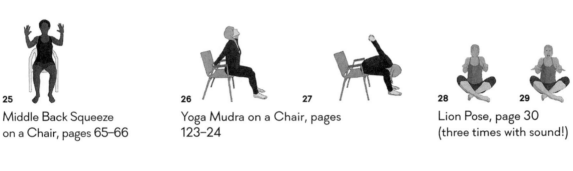

25 **26** **27** **28** **29**

Middle Back Squeeze on a Chair, pages 65–66

Yoga Mudra on a Chair, pages 123–24

Lion Pose, page 30 (three times with sound!)

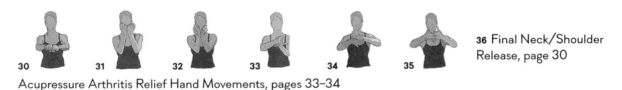

30 **31** **32** **33** **34** **35** **36** Final Neck/Shoulder Release, page 30

Acupressure Arthritis Relief Hand Movements, pages 33–34

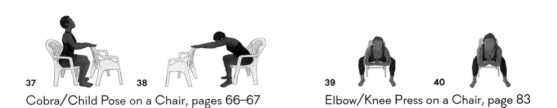

37 **38** **39** **40**

Cobra/Child Pose on a Chair, pages 66–67

Elbow/Knee Press on a Chair, page 83

continues on next page

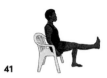

41
Leg Raises on a Chair, pages 67–68

42
Seated Backward Bend on a Chair, page 69

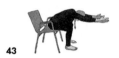

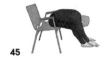

43 **44** **45**

Seated Forward Bends on a Chair, pages 122–23
(do all or choose variations)

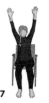
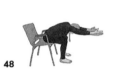

46 **47** **48** **49** **50** **51**

Sun Salutation Series on a Chair, pages 124–27 (three rounds)

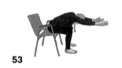

52 **53** **54** **55** **56**

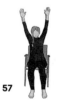

57 **58**

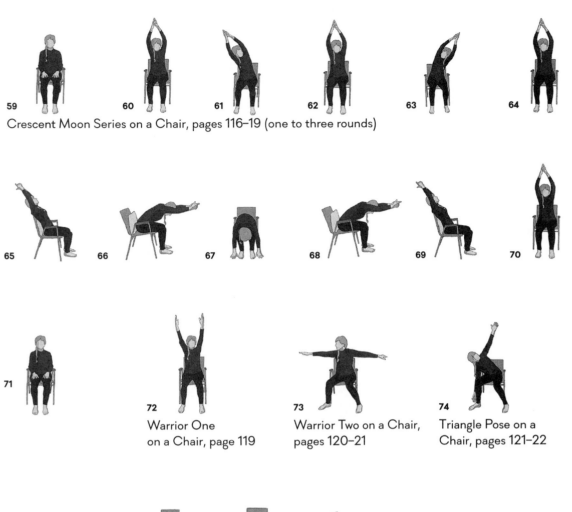

Crescent Moon Series on a Chair, pages 116–19 (one to three rounds)

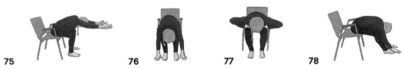

72 Warrior One on a Chair, page 119

73 Warrior Two on a Chair, pages 120–21

74 Triangle Pose on a Chair, pages 121–22

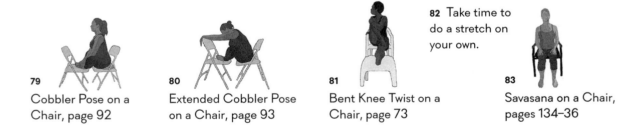

Repeat Seated Forward Bends on a Chair, pages 122–23 (do all or choose one variation)

79 Cobbler Pose on a Chair, page 92

80 Extended Cobbler Pose on a Chair, page 93

81 Bent Knee Twist on a Chair, page 73

82 Take time to do a stretch on your own.

83 Savasana on a Chair, pages 134–36

Sequence for Shoulders/Neck on a Mat

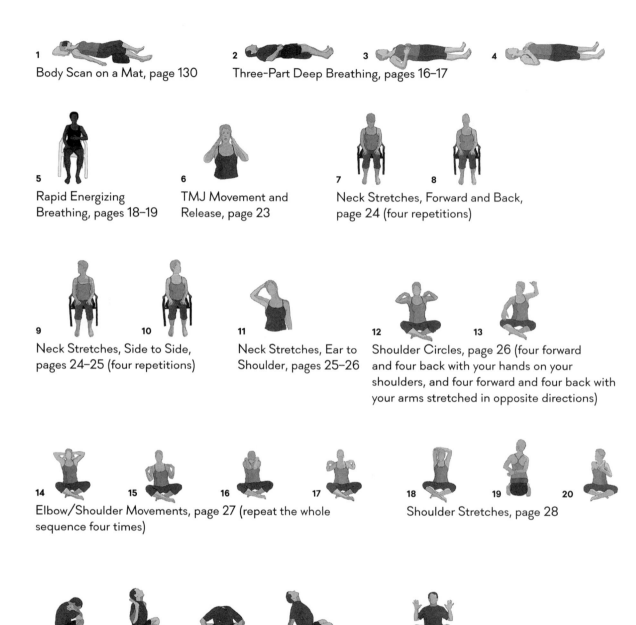

1 Body Scan on a Mat, page 130

2 3 4 Three-Part Deep Breathing, pages 16–17

5 Rapid Energizing Breathing, pages 18–19

6 TMJ Movement and Release, page 23

7 8 Neck Stretches, Forward and Back, page 24 (four repetitions)

9 10 Neck Stretches, Side to Side, pages 24–25 (four repetitions)

11 Neck Stretches, Ear to Shoulder, pages 25–26

12 13 Shoulder Circles, page 26 (four forward and four back with your hands on your shoulders, and four forward and four back with your arms stretched in opposite directions)

14 15 16 17 Elbow/Shoulder Movements, page 27 (repeat the whole sequence four times)

18 19 20 Shoulder Stretches, page 28

21 22 23 24 Rounding and Arching on a Mat, pages 38–39

25 Middle Back Squeeze on a Mat, page 39

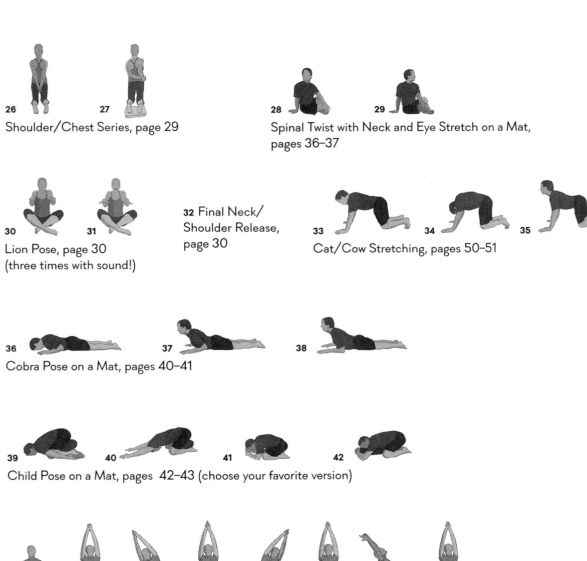

26 **27** Shoulder/Chest Series, page 29

28 **29** Spinal Twist with Neck and Eye Stretch on a Mat, pages 36–37

30 **31** Lion Pose, page 30 (three times with sound!)

32 Final Neck/ Shoulder Release, page 30

33 **34** **35** Cat/Cow Stretching, pages 50–51

36 **37** **38** Cobra Pose on a Mat, pages 40–41

39 **40** **41** **42** Child Pose on a Mat, pages 42–43 (choose your favorite version)

43 **44** **45** **46** **47** **48** **49** **50** Standing Crescent Moon Series, pages 98–100

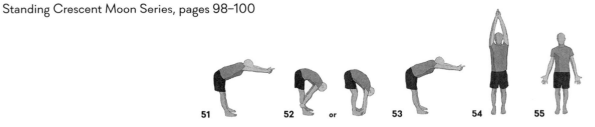

51 **52** or **53** **54** **55**

continues on next page

56 Standing Warrior One, pages 100–101

57 Standing Warrior Two, pages 101–3

58 Standing Triangle Pose, pages 103–4

59 Standing Yoga Mudra, pages 106–7

60

61 Take time to do a stretch on your own.

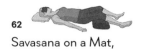

62 Savasana on a Mat, pages 131–34

SEQUENCE FOR SHOULDERS/NECK ON A CHAIR

(Two sturdy chairs are needed for this sequence)

1 Body Scan, page 130

2 Three-Part Deep Breathing, pages 16–17

3 Rapid Energizing Breathing, pages 18–19

4 TMJ Movement and Release, page 23

5 **6** Neck Stretches, Forward and Back, page 24 (four repetitions)

7 **8** Neck Stretches, Side to Side, pages 24–25 (four repetitions)

9 Neck Stretches, Ear to Shoulder, pages 25–26

10 **11** Shoulder Circles, page 26 (four forward and four back with your hands on your shoulders, and four forward and four back with your arms stretched in opposite directions)

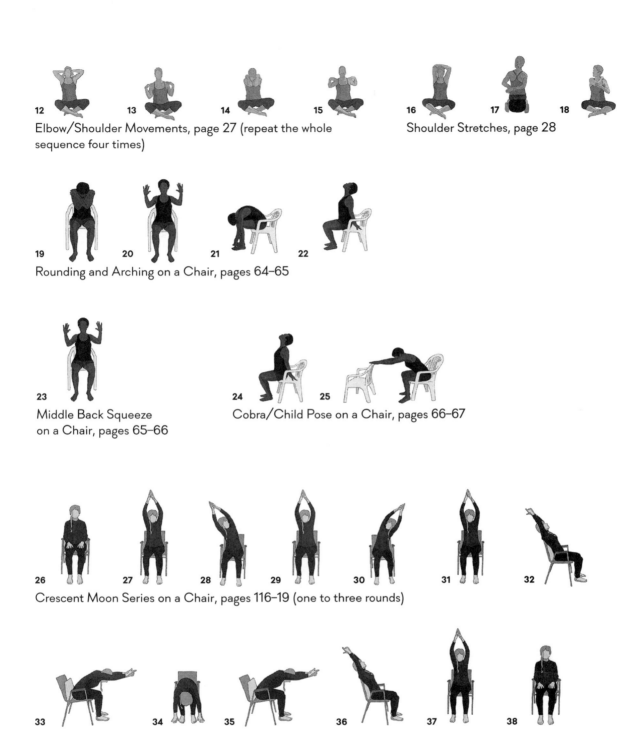

12 **13** **14** **15**   **16** **17** **18**

Elbow/Shoulder Movements, page 27 (repeat the whole sequence four times)   Shoulder Stretches, page 28

19 **20** **21** **22**

Rounding and Arching on a Chair, pages 64–65

23

Middle Back Squeeze on a Chair, pages 65–66   **24** **25**   Cobra/Child Pose on a Chair, pages 66–67

26 **27** **28** **29** **30** **31** **32**

Crescent Moon Series on a Chair, pages 116–19 (one to three rounds)

33 **34** **35** **36** **37** **38**

continues on next page

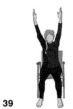

39
Warrior One
on a Chair, page 119

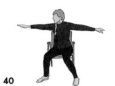

40
Warrior Two on a Chair,
pages 120–21

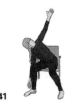

41
Triangle Pose on a
Chair, pages 121–22

42

43
Yoga Mudra on a Chair, pages 123–24

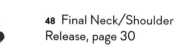

44

45
Spinal Twist with Neck and Eye Stretch on a Chair,
pages 62–63 (with knees to the side if necessary)

46

47
Lion Pose, page 30
(three times with sound!)

48 Final Neck/Shoulder
Release, page 30

49 Take time to do a
stretch on your own.

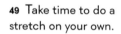

50
Savasana on a Chair, pages 134–36

SEQUENCE FOR LOWER BACK ON A MAT

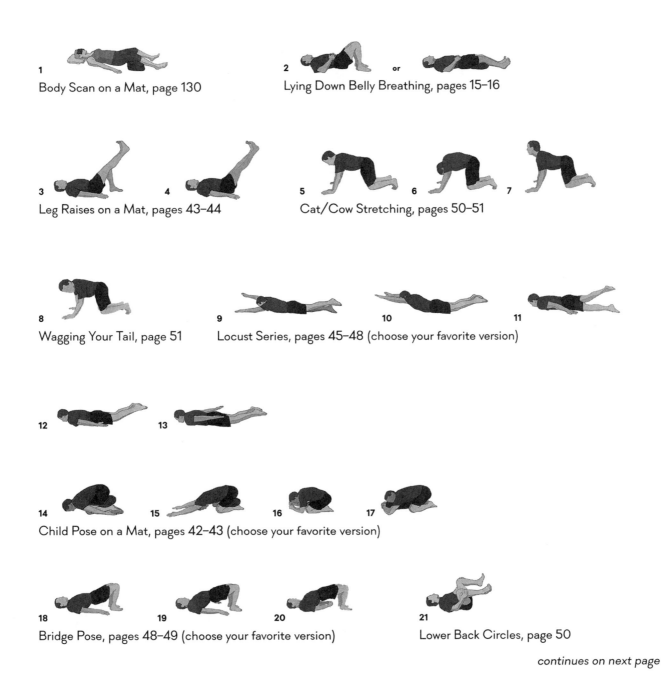

1
Body Scan on a Mat, page 130

2 or
Lying Down Belly Breathing, pages 15–16

3 **4**
Leg Raises on a Mat, pages 43–44

5 **6** **7**
Cat/Cow Stretching, pages 50–51

8
Wagging Your Tail, page 51

9 **10** **11**
Locust Series, pages 45–48 (choose your favorite version)

12 **13**

14 **15** **16** **17**
Child Pose on a Mat, pages 42–43 (choose your favorite version)

18 **19** **20**
Bridge Pose, pages 48–49 (choose your favorite version)

21
Lower Back Circles, page 50

continues on next page

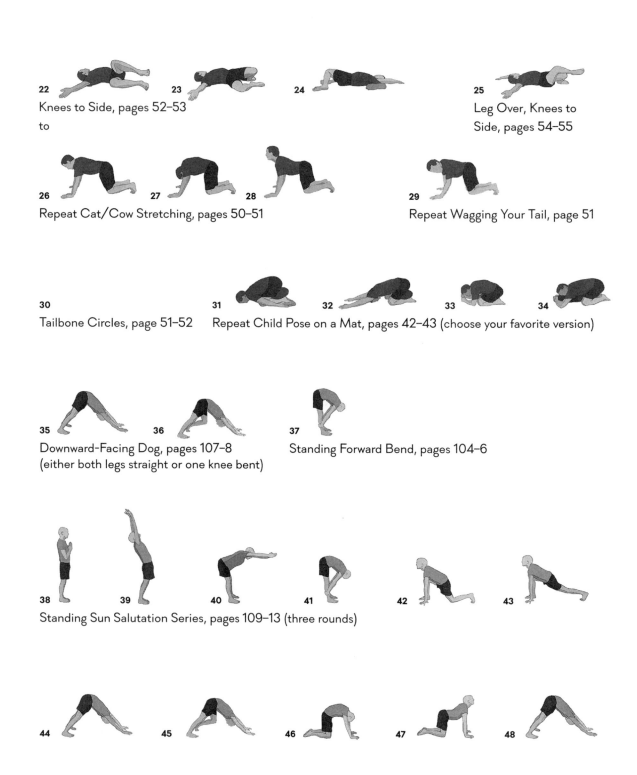

22
23
24
25

Knees to Side, pages 52–53
to

Leg Over, Knees to
Side, pages 54–55

26
27
28
29

Repeat Cat/Cow Stretching, pages 50–51

Repeat Wagging Your Tail, page 51

30
31
32
33
34

Tailbone Circles, page 51–52
Repeat Child Pose on a Mat, pages 42–43 (choose your favorite version)

35
36
37

Downward-Facing Dog, pages 107–8
(either both legs straight or one knee bent)
Standing Forward Bend, pages 104–6

38
39
40
41
42
43

Standing Sun Salutation Series, pages 109–13 (three rounds)

44
45
46
47
48

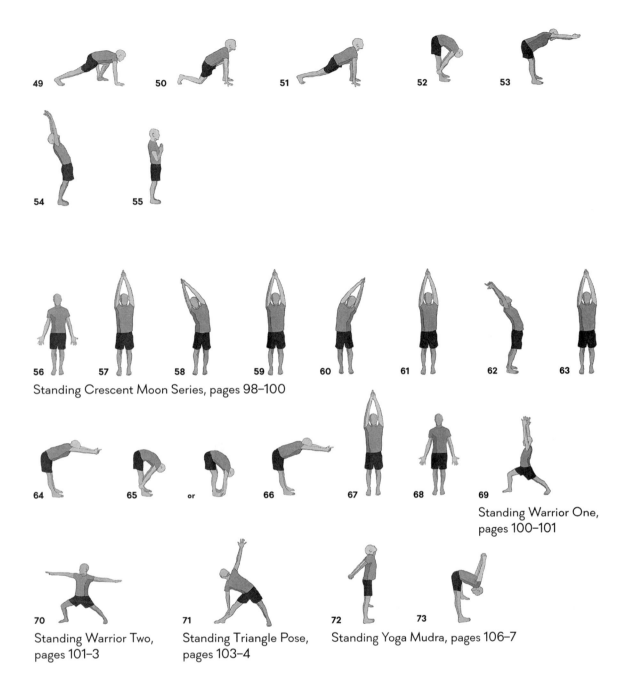

Standing Crescent Moon Series, pages 98–100

Standing Warrior One,
pages 100–101

Standing Warrior Two,
pages 101–3

Standing Triangle Pose,
pages 103–4

Standing Yoga Mudra, pages 106–7

continues on next page

74
Repeat Standing Forward
Bend, pages 104–6

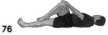 **75** 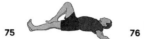 **76** 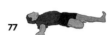 **77**
Knee Down Twist (last part of the Hip-Stretching Sequence), page 58

 78 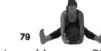 **79** 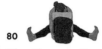 **80** **81** Take time to do a
stretch on your own. 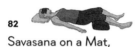 **82**
Full Forward Bend on a Mat, page 89 (with either a belt or a bolster) Savasana on a Mat,
pages 131–34

SEQUENCE FOR LOWER BACK ON A CHAIR

(Two sturdy chairs are needed for this sequence)

 1
Body Scan, page 130 **2**
Seated Belly
Breathing,
pages 14–15 **3** **4** **5** **6**
Rounding and Arching on a Chair, pages 64–65

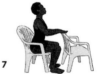 **7** 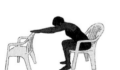 **8**
Cobra/Child Pose on a Chair, pages 66–67 **9**
Leg Raises
on a Chair, pages
67–68 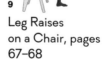 **10**
Seated Backward Bend
on a Chair, page 69

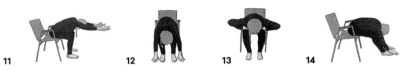

Seated Forward Bends on a Chair, pages 122–23 (do all or choose one variation)

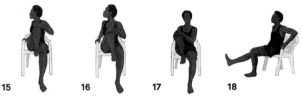

Hip-Stretching Sequence on a Chair, pages 69–71

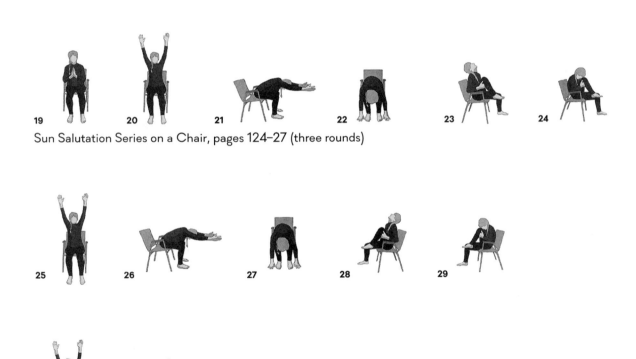

Sun Salutation Series on a Chair, pages 124–27 (three rounds)

continues on next page

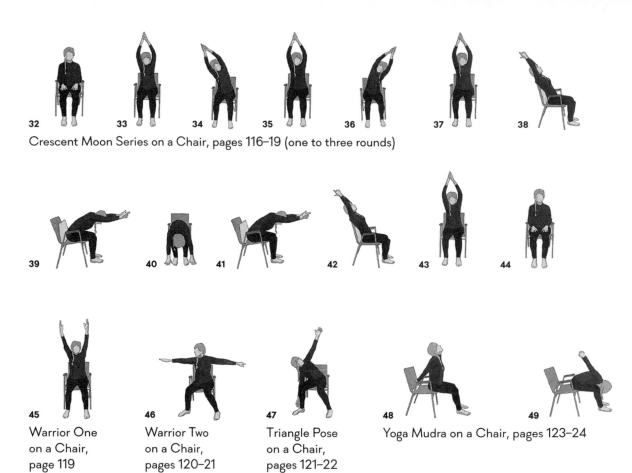

Crescent Moon Series on a Chair, pages 116–19 (one to three rounds)

Warrior One on a Chair, page 119

Warrior Two on a Chair, pages 120–21

Triangle Pose on a Chair, pages 121–22

Yoga Mudra on a Chair, pages 123–24

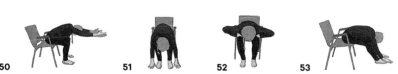

Repeat Seated Forward Bends on a Chair, pages 122–23 (do all or choose one variation)

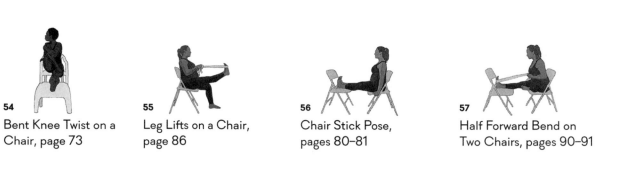

Bent Knee Twist on a Chair, page 73

Leg Lifts on a Chair, page 86

Chair Stick Pose, pages 80–81

Half Forward Bend on Two Chairs, pages 90–91

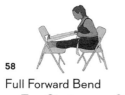

58 Full Forward Bend on Two Chairs, page 91

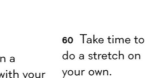

59 Simple Spinal Twist on a Chair, pages 61–62 (with your knees to the side if necessary)

60 Take time to do a stretch on your own.

61 Savasana on a Chair, pages 134–36

SEQUENCE FOR HIPS ON A MAT

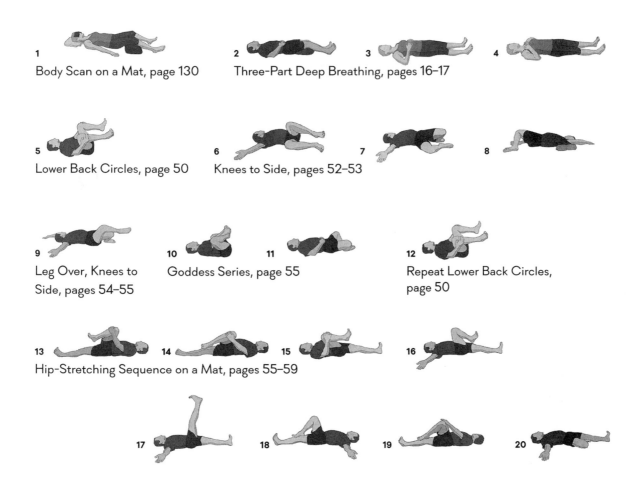

1 Body Scan on a Mat, page 130

2 **3** **4** Three-Part Deep Breathing, pages 16–17

5 Lower Back Circles, page 50

6 **7** **8** Knees to Side, pages 52–53

9 Leg Over, Knees to Side, pages 54–55

10 **11** Goddess Series, page 55

12 Repeat Lower Back Circles, page 50

13 **14** **15** **16** Hip-Stretching Sequence on a Mat, pages 55–59

17 **18** **19** **20**

continues on next page

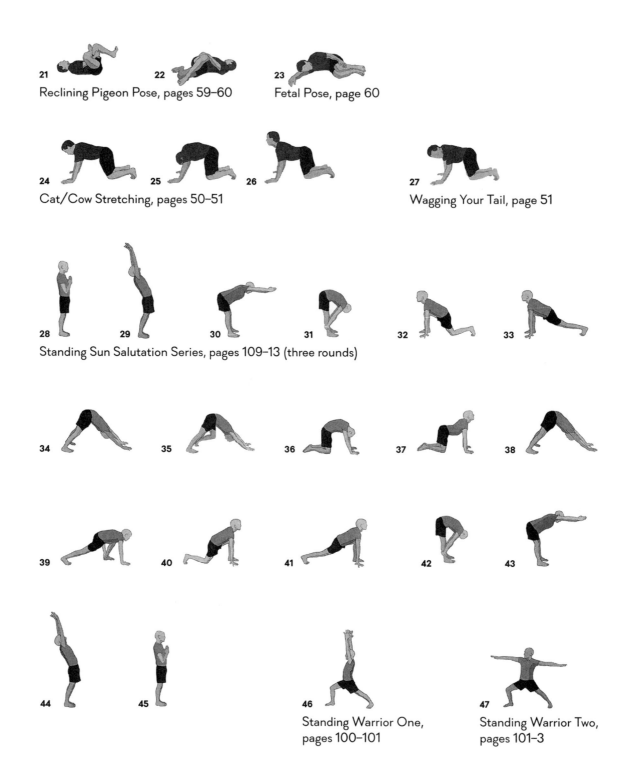

21 **22** **23**
Reclining Pigeon Pose, pages 59–60   Fetal Pose, page 60

24 **25** **26** **27**
Cat/Cow Stretching, pages 50–51   Wagging Your Tail, page 51

28 **29** **30** **31** **32** **33**
Standing Sun Salutation Series, pages 109–13 (three rounds)

34 **35** **36** **37** **38**

39 **40** **41** **42** **43**

44 **45** **46** **47**
Standing Warrior One, pages 100–101   Standing Warrior Two, pages 101–3

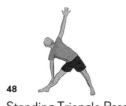

48
Standing Triangle Pose,
pages 103–4

49 **50**
Standing Yoga Mudra, pages 106–7

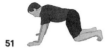 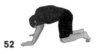 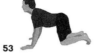 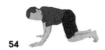

51 **52** **53**
Repeat Cat/Cow Stretching, pages 50–51

54
Repeat Wagging Your Tail, page 51

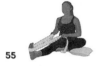 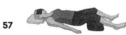

55
Half Forward Bend
on a Mat, page 88

56 Take time to do a
stretch on your own.

57
Savasana on a Mat,
pages 131–34

Sequence for Hips on a Chair

(Two sturdy chairs are needed for this sequence)

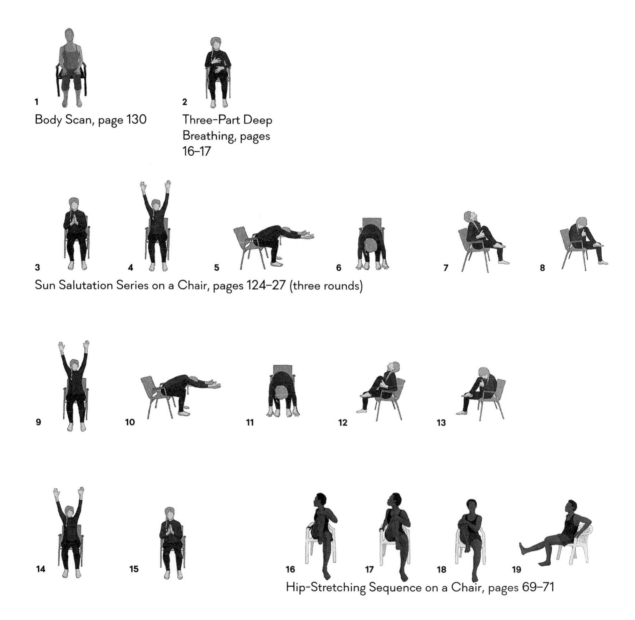

1

Body Scan, page 130

2

Three-Part Deep Breathing, pages 16–17

Sun Salutation Series on a Chair, pages 124–27 (three rounds)

3 **4** **5** **6** **7** **8**

9 **10** **11** **12** **13**

14 **15** **16** **17** **18** **19**

Hip-Stretching Sequence on a Chair, pages 69–71

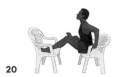

20
Pigeon Pose on Two
Chairs, pages 71–72

21

22
Bent Knee Twist on a Chair, page 73

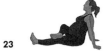

23
Knee/Hip/Ankle Warm Up,
page 76

24
Leg Cradling, page 77

25
Bent Knee Circling,
page 77

26

27
Elbow/Knee Press on a Chair, page 83

28
Leg Lifts on a Chair,
page 86

29
Leg Lifts to the Side on a Chair,
page 87

30

31
Half Forward Bend on Two
Chairs, pages 90–91

32
Cobbler Pose on a Chair,
page 92

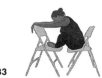

33
Extended Cobbler Pose
on a Chair, page 93

34 Take time to
do a stretch on
your own.

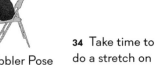

35
Savasana on a Chair,
pages 134–36

Sequence for Legs, Knees, Ankles, and Feet on a Mat

1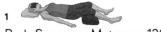
Body Scan on a Mat, page 130

2 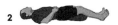 **3** 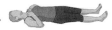 **4**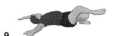
Three-Part Deep Breathing, pages 16–17

5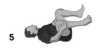
Lower Back Circles, page 50

6 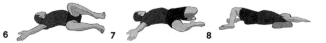 **7** **8** **9**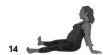
Knees to Side, pages 52–53

Leg Over, Knees to Side, pages 54–55

10 **11** **12** 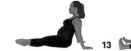 **13** **14**
Stick Pose, pages 80–81

Foot Stretches, pages 81–82

15 **16** **17** **18** **19** **20**
Isometric Foot Press, pages 82–83

Elbow/Knee Press on a Mat, page 83

Acupressure Knee-Strengthening Exercise, pages 79–80

21 **22** **23** 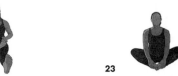 **24**
Foot/Leg Massage, page 78

Cobbler Pose on a Mat, page 92

Extended Cobbler Pose on a Mat, page 93

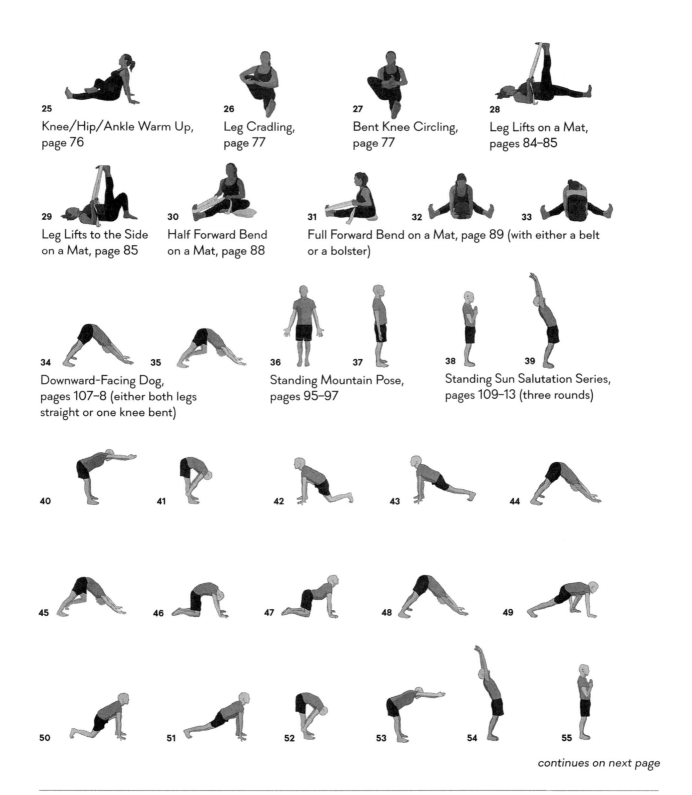

25 Knee/Hip/Ankle Warm Up, page 76

26 Leg Cradling, page 77

27 Bent Knee Circling, page 77

28 Leg Lifts on a Mat, pages 84–85

29 Leg Lifts to the Side on a Mat, page 85

30 Half Forward Bend on a Mat, page 88

31 **32** **33** Full Forward Bend on a Mat, page 89 (with either a belt or a bolster)

34 **35** Downward-Facing Dog, pages 107–8 (either both legs straight or one knee bent)

36 **37** Standing Mountain Pose, pages 95–97

38 **39** Standing Sun Salutation Series, pages 109–13 (three rounds)

40

41

42

43

44

45

46

47

48

49

50

51

52

53

54

55

continues on next page

56
Standing Warrior One,
pages 100–101

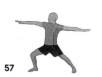
57
Standing Warrior Two,
pages 101–3

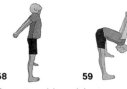
58　　　**59**
Standing Yoga Mudra,
pages 106–7

60
Standing Forward
Bend, pages 104–6

61　　　**62**
Reclining Pigeon Pose, pages 59–60

63　　　**64**
Goddess Series, page 55

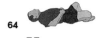
65
Lower Back Circles,
page 50

66 Take time to do a
stretch on your own.

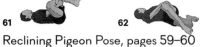
67
Savasana on a Mat,
pages 131–34

SEQUENCE FOR LEGS, KNEES, ANKLES, AND FEET ON A CHAIR

(Two sturdy chairs are needed for this sequence)

1
Body Scan, page 130

2
Three-Part Deep
Breathing, pages
16–17

3
Leg Raises on a Chair,
pages 67–68

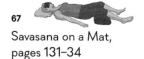

4　　　**5**　　　**6**　　　**7**
Hip-Stretching Sequence on a Chair, pages 69–71

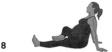
8
Knee/Hip/Ankle Warm Up, page 76

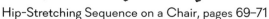

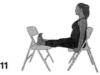

9
10
11

Leg Cradling,
page 77

Bent Knee Circling,
page 77

Chair Stick Pose,
pages 80–81

 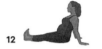 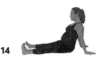 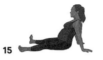

12
13
14
15
16

Foot Stretches, pages 81–82

Isometric Foot Press,
pages 82–83

 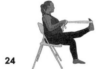

17
18
19
20
21

Elbow/Knee Press on a Chair, page 83

Acupressure Knee-Strengthening Exercise, pages 79–80

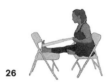   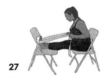

22
23
24
25

Foot/Leg Massage, page 78

Leg Lifts on a Chair,
page 86

Leg Lifts to the Side
on a Chair, page 87

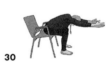

26
27
28
29
30

Half Forward Bend
on Two Chairs, pages
90–91

Full Forward Bend on Two
Chairs, page 91

Sun Salutation Series on a Chair, pages 124–27
(three rounds)

continues on next page

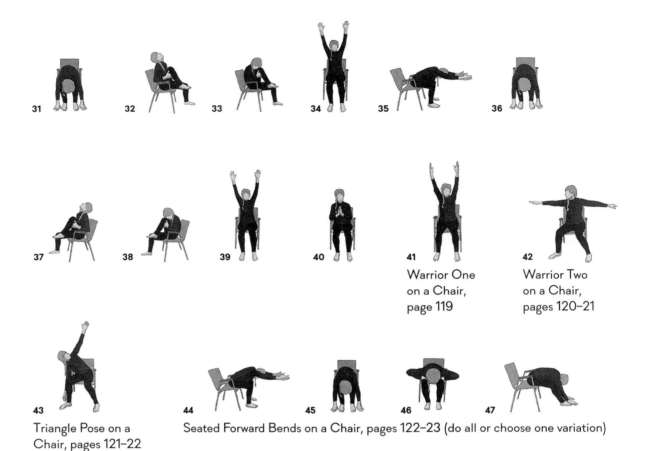

31 **32** **33** **34** **35** **36**

37 **38** **39** **40**

41 Warrior One on a Chair, page 119

42 Warrior Two on a Chair, pages 120–21

43 Triangle Pose on a Chair, pages 121–22

44 **45** **46** **47** Seated Forward Bends on a Chair, pages 122–23 (do all or choose one variation)

48 Pigeon Pose on Two Chairs, page 71–72

49 **50** Bent Knee Twist on a Chair, page 73

51 Cobbler Pose on a Chair, page 92

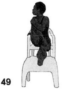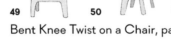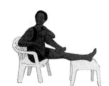

52 Extended Cobbler Pose on a Chair, page 93

53 Take time to do a stretch on your own.

54 Savasana on a Chair, pages 134–36

Acknowledgments

I WANT TO THANK Josh Bartok, my Zen friend, teacher, and Wisdom Publications editor, who called me in 2009 and suggested I write this book. He said, "It will be an easy and fun book to write." It wasn't always easy, but it was fun and I am so grateful to have had the opportunity to pour out all this stuff I have been holding in my brain for forty years. I offer deep gratitude to Laura Cunningham, Wisdom editor, who was always available with guidance, kind words, and encouragement as she kept me on track. I offer a bow to Michelle Antonisse for her gorgeous illustrations and her patience in explaining over and over how we could get the photos right (as well as her expertise in fixing the ones we never did get right).

I have much appreciation for my dear friends Susie Patlove (Zen meditator and writer), Ellen Kaufmann (physical therapist), and Eowyn Ahlstrom (meditator/yogini), all of whom read the book at different stages and gave me honest, professional feedback. I want to recognize the many years of inspiration, love, and support I have received from the past and present codirectors—Libby Volckening, Marilyn Mullen, and Anna Meyer—and the students at Green River Yoga Center in Greenfield, MA. I honor my Zen teachers (Josh Bartok, Melissa Blacker, James Ford, and David Rynick) and my beloved Boundless Way Zen sangha, who taught me how best to lead worn-out meditators in gentle yoga stretches. I honor all my yoga teachers, especially Bonnie Bainbridge Cohen and Lakshmi Voelker, both of whom allowed me to include their wisdom in this book.

I am blessed by an immediate and extended family who cheered me on and only complained a little that I spent too much time at the computer over the past few years: Anna Erlbaum-Rumelt, Libby Erlbaum-Rumelt, Evan Becker, Mo Jones, Amy Rumelt, Paul Erlbaum, Rachael Grossman, Lynne Schachne, Susan Mailler, Dale Schwarz, Guillermo

Cuellar, Karen Brandow, Linda Marchesani, Carol Drexler, and my very special aunt Adele Kimowitz (1919–2012), who took me to my first yoga class in 1965!

This book would not have happened without the generosity and patience of all the models: Kathi Batsis, Mo Jones, Gary Newcomb, Ari Pliskin, Sojee Raymond, and Amy Rumelt (each of whom have a brief bio at the end of this book).

My husband and best friend, Richard Rumelt, did an amazing job of taking all the photographs of those models. He gave up hours of his newly retired life putting up with me, Laura, and Michelle giving more and more detailed directions on how to best take the pictures. Richie has supported me throughout a lifetime of doing what I love most. Together we have raised two amazing daughters and now, together, we have created this book. I am so grateful for his love and our partnership.

Suggested Resources

BOOKS

Anderson, Bob, and Jean Anderson. *Stretching: 30th Anniversary Edition.* Bolinas, California: Shelter Publications, 2010.

Boccio, Frank Jude. *Mindfulness Yoga.* Boston: Wisdom Publications, 2004.

Cappy, Peggy. *Yoga for All of Us.* New York: St. Martin's Griffin, 2006.

Cohen, Bonnie Bainbridge. *Sensing, Feeling, and Action.* 2nd ed. El Sobrante, CA: Birchfield Rose, 2008.

Friedman, Lenore, and Susan Moon. *Being Bodies: Buddhist Women on the Paradox of Embodiment.* Boston and New York: Shambhala, 1997.

Kerr, Meera Patricia. *Big Yoga, A Simple Guide for Bigger Bodies.* New York: Square One Publishers, 2010.

Lee, Cyndi. *Yoga Body, Buddha Mind.* New York: Riverhead Books, 2004.

Lincoln, Jerri. *Wheelchair Yoga.* Durango, CO: Ralston Store Publishing, 2012.

Noble, Elizabeth. *Essential Exercises for the Childbearing Year.* 4th ed. Harwich, MA: New Life Images, 2003.

Schaeffer, Rachel. *Yoga for Your Spiritual Muscles.* Wheaton, IL: Quest Books, 1998.

Schatz, Mary Pullig, MD. *Back Care Basics.* Berkeley, CA: Rodmell Press, 1992.

Schiffmann, Erich. *Yoga: The Spirit and Practice of Moving into Stillness.* New York: Pocket Books, 1996.

CDS/DVDS

For information about companion CDs for *Sit with Less Pain: Gentle Yoga for Meditators and Everyone Else*, please contact the author at jean.erlbaum@verizon.net or info@sitwithlesspain.com, www.sitwithlesspain.com.

Anderson, Bob. *Stretching.* (DVD)

Cappy, Peggy. *Yoga for the Rest of Us with Peggy Cappy.* (DVD)

Cappy, Peggy. *Yoga for the Rest of Us— Back Care Basics.* (DVD)

Erlbaum, Jean. *Yoga for Relaxation.* (Two gentle yoga classes on CD)

Voelker, Lakshmi. *Single Chair Yoga, vol. 1.* (DVD)

Voelker, Lakshmi. *The Sitting Mountain Series Audio CD and Tutorial Booklet.*

WEBSITES

www.bodymindcentering.com (Bonnie Bainbridge Cohen information and resources)

www.getfitwhereyousit.com (Lakshmi Voelker's Chair Yoga)

www.peggycappy.net

www.sitwithlesspain.com (book information and companion CDs for *Sit with Less Pain: Gentle Yoga for Meditators and Everyone Else*)

www.yogaforrelaxation.org (Jean Erlbaum's classes and CDs)

About the Contributors

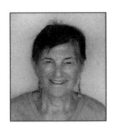

JEAN ERLBAUM, MS, ERYT, LVCYT, has been studying yoga and meditation since 1965 and has been teaching since 1972. An Experienced Registered 500-Hour Yoga Teacher, she is certified as a teacher of several styles of yoga, meditation, and stress reduction. She has studied Zen for over thirty years and in 2012 was designated as a senior Dharma teacher by Boundless Way Zen (Worcester, MA). She offers classes in Greenfield, MA, and Naples, FL, where she lives with her husband Richard Rumelt and their two daschunds, Stella and Oscar. Richard and Jean have two daughters, Anna and Libby, who live in New York City. For more information about Jean, her classes, and media resources, please go 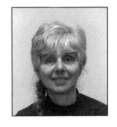 to www.yogaforrelaxation.org or www.sitwithlesspain.com.

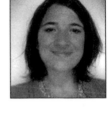

MICHELLE ANTONISSE, illustrator, is an artist living in Los Angeles and an educator at the Museum of Contemporary Art. Her previous illustration work includes *Veggiyana: The Dharma of Cooking* (Wisdom Publications, 2011).

KATHI BATSIS (model for "Standing Poses: Variations for Chair") is enjoying her retirement, which is filled with writing, knitting, tai chi, scrabble, dancing, singing, and learning French. She taught herself yoga from Richard Hittleman's book in 1975 and is now a member of Jeanie Erlbaum's Over 50 Yoga class in Greenfield, MA.

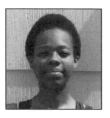

Mo Jones (model for "Mid-Body: Variations for a Chair") is a new practitioner of yoga. Her life passions are photography and cooking. She currently works as a lead line cook in New York City.

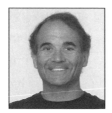

Gary Newcomb (model for "Mid-Body") is a certified Iyengar Yoga instructor from Greenfield, MA. He has been an avid competitive athlete for over thirty-five years in track and field, martial arts, and swimming and has been practicing yoga for thirty years.

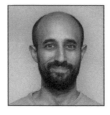

Ari Pliskin (model for "Standing Poses") is a Zen yogi who enjoys spiritual practice on the streets as much as on the mat. Under the auspices of the Zen Peacemakers, he helped create and continues to manage the Stone Soup

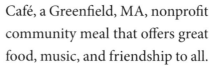

Café, a Greenfield, MA, nonprofit community meal that offers great food, music, and friendship to all.

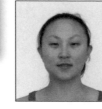

Sojee Raymond (model for "Legs, Knees, Ankles, and Feet") is a well-loved massage therapist in Greenfield, MA. Her beautiful daughter, Millena Tansy Strom, was born November 18, 2012, about a month after she finished posing for this book.

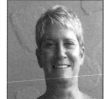

Amy Rumelt (model for "Upper Body") is newly retired after twenty years of having been a teacher and then the principal of a school for students with special needs. Besides being an enthusiastic yogini, she enjoys motorscooters, digital photography, and reading mysteries while sitting by the pool at her new home in Naples, Florida.

About Wisdom Publications

WISDOM PUBLICATIONS is the leading publisher of contemporary and classic Buddhist books and practical works on mindfulness. Publishing books from all major Buddhist traditions, Wisdom is a nonprofit charitable organization dedicated to cultivating Buddhist voices the world over, advancing critical scholarship, and preserving and sharing Buddhist literary culture.

To learn more about us or to explore our other books, please visit our website at www .wisdompubs.org. You can subscribe to our eNewsletter, request a print catalog, and find out how you can help support Wisdom's mission either online or by writing to:

Wisdom Publications
199 Elm Street
Somerville, Massachusetts 02144 USA

You can also contact us at 617-776-7416, or info@wisdompubs.org.

Wisdom is a 501(c)(3) organization, and donations in support of our mission are tax deductible.

Wisdom Publications is affiliated with the Foundation for the Preservation of the Mahayana Tradition (FPMT).

Also Available from Wisdom Publications

Mindfulness Yoga

The Awakened Union of Breath, Body, and Mind

Frank Jude Boccio

368 pages | 8.25 x 10″ | $19.95

9780861713356 | 9780861719754

"EDITOR'S CHOICE!
Boccio shows that Buddhist practice is itself a form of yoga,
presenting a meditational approach to asana practice."
—*Yoga Journal*

Veggiyana

The Dharma of Cooking: With 108 Deliciously Easy Vegetarian Recipes

Sandra Garson

320 pages | 7 x 10" | $19.95

9780861716364 | 9780861718818

"*Veggiyana* is more than just a cookbook—it's a feast in itself. It is a book to be
treasured, living as it will in my kitchen and in my heart."
—Toni Bernhard, author of *How to Be Sick:
A Buddhist-Inspired Guide for the Chronically Ill and Their Caregivers*